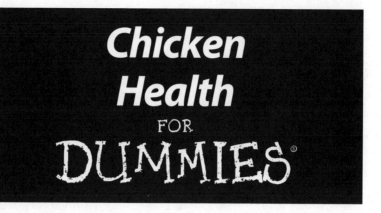

Chicken Health

FOR

DUMMIES®

by Julie Gauthier, DVM, MPH, Dipl. ACVPM, and Rob Ludlow

D1354922

WILEY

John Wiley & Sons, Inc.

Chicken Health For Dummies®

Published by
John Wiley & Sons, Inc.
111 River St.
Hoboken, NJ 07030-5774
www.wiley.com

Copyright © 2013 by John Wiley & Sons, Inc., Hoboken, New Jersey

Published by John Wiley & Sons, Inc., Hoboken, New Jersey

Published simultaneously in Canada

For general information on our other products and services, please contact our Customer Care Department within the U.S. at 877-762-2974, outside the U.S. at 317-572-3993, or fax 317-572-4002.

For technical support, please visit www.wiley.com/techsupport.

Wiley publishes in a variety of print and electronic formats and by print-on-demand. Some material included with standard print versions of this book may not be included in e-books or in print-on-demand. If this book refers to media such as a CD or DVD that is not included in the version you purchased, you may download this material at http://booksupport.wiley.com. For more information about Wiley products, visit www.wiley.com.

Library of Congress Control Number: 2012954765

ISBN 978-1-118-44427-6 (pbk); ISBN 978-1-118-46096-2 (ebk); ISBN 978-1-118-46097-9 (ebk); 978-1-118-46098-6 (ebk)

Manufactured in the United States of America

10 9 8 7 6 5 4

WILEY

About the Authors

Julie Gauthier graduated from veterinary school at Michigan State University in 1993, earned a master's degree in public health from Yale University in 2002, and became board certified in veterinary preventive medicine in 2009. Julie practiced large and small animal medicine for nine years in three different states; during that time, her favorite patients were chickens. Joining the USDA Animal and Plant Health Inspection Service in 2002 gave Julie the opportunity to see all kinds of flocks, great and small, all over the world, in her work as a veterinary epidemiologist (an animal disease detective). On her small farm in North Carolina, Julie raises heritage breed chickens, ducks, and turkeys for exhibition, good food, and conservation of these vanishing breeds.

Rob Ludlow owns and manages www.BackYardChickens.com (BYC), the largest and fastest growing community of chicken enthusiasts in the world. Rob is also the co-author of the books *Raising Chickens For Dummies* and *Building Chicken Coops For Dummies* (John Wiley & Sons, Inc.).

Rob, his wife Emily, and their two beautiful daughters, Alana and April, are the perfect example of the suburban family with a small flock of backyard chickens. Like countless others, what started out as a fun hobby raising a few egg-laying machines has almost turned into an addiction.

Dedication

From Julie: To my family, Kenna, Garret, and Mark, who picked up the slack on the poultry chores.

From Rob: To the many wonderful chickens that have been part of our flock-family over the years including Goldie, Blackie, Blackie-Whitey, Whitey, Reddy, Cleo, Lilly, Sparkles, and especially Ginger!

Authors' Acknowledgments

From Julie: I want to send out a crow of thanks to my brother, Dr. Dave Gauthier, for photographing deconstructed feathered creatures (rather than his usual finned subjects) on one hot summer day. To my flock mates I.K., S.K., M.M., S.L, W.C., and J.L.: I'll express my thanks for your encouragement, support, and enthusiasm by saving the biggest, juiciest worms for you. Thanks also to Ms. Elizabeth Clark and Dr. Tahseen Aziz for contributing excellent photographs, and being just as intrigued as I am by cyanotic combs and torticollis. I sincerely appreciate the professionalism, skill, and good nature shown to me by staff of Wiley, especially Alissa Schwipps, Erin Calligan Mooney, Chad Sievers, David Hobson, and the Wiley Composition team. Our intrepid and patient illustrators Kathryn Born and Barbara Frake deserve an appreciative cackle, too. Best regards to my friends of the Delaware Poultry Club, the Triangle Area Gardeners and Homesteaders, and the American Livestock Breeds Conservancy; thanks for giving me my start as a flock keeper self-help coach.

From Rob: A ton of appreciation and love to the countless members of BackYardChickens.com, and especially the BYC moderators who have collectively (and patiently) educated me over the years. Thanks to the team at Wiley for all their amazing work, patience, expertise, and diligence, especially that from Erin Calligan Mooney, Alissa Schwipps, and David Hobson.

Publisher's Acknowledgments

We're proud of this book; please send us your comments at `http://dummies.custhelp.com`. For other comments, please contact our Customer Care Department within the U.S. at 877-762-2974, outside the U.S. at 317-572-3993, or fax 317-572-4002.

Some of the people who helped bring this book to market include the following:

Acquisitions, Editorial, and Vertical Websites

Senior Project Editor: Alissa Schwipps

Acquisitions Editor: Erin Calligan Mooney

Copy Editor: Chad R. Sievers

Assistant Editor: David Lutton

Editorial Program Coordinator: Joe Niesen

Technical Editor: Teresa Y. Morishita, DVM, PhD, Dipl. ACPV

Editorial Manager: Christine Meloy Beck

Editorial Assistants: Rachelle S. Amick, Alexa Koschier

Art Coordinator: Alicia B. South

Cover Photo: ©Chelsea Fuss / Getty Images

Cartoons: Rich Tennant (`www.the5thwave.com`)

Composition Services

Project Coordinator: Sheree Montgomery

Layout and Graphics: Jennifer Creasey, Brent Savage

Proofreader: Judith Q. McMullen

Indexer: BIM Indexing & Proofreading Services

Illustrators: Kathryn Born, Barbara Frake

Publishing and Editorial for Consumer Dummies

> **Kathleen Nebenhaus,** Vice President and Executive Publisher

> **David Palmer,** Associate Publisher

> **Kristin Ferguson-Wagstaffe,** Product Development Director

Publishing for Technology Dummies

> **Andy Cummings,** Vice President and Publisher

Composition Services

> **Debbie Stailey,** Director of Composition Services

Contents at a Glance

Table of Contents

Introduction

● ●

*W*elcome to *Chicken Health For Dummies*. If you want to
know practical ways to keep a small flock healthy, or know
what to do when a backyard chicken is ill or injured, this book is
for you.

At this point in your chicken-keeping career, more than likely,
you're already (or you're about to become) thoroughly hooked on
the freshest of eggs, you're perpetually surprised by the voracious
curiosity of your foraging flock, and you're up-to-date with the soap
opera of the hen house. Along with the joys of raising chickens,
though, you (or one of your flock-keeping friends) probably have
experienced at least one disappointment: a devastating predator
attack, a droopy chick, or the horrifying discovery that the gorgeous
hen you picked up at the swap meet is crawling with lice.

We've been there, and dealt with that, and we want to share our
experiences — joyful and dismaying — to help you fly through the
challenges of caring for your flock. In these pages, we have something for everyone, from wanna-be flock keepers to old hands, and
from high-rise rooftop farmers to people at home on the range.

About This Book

We want *Chicken Health For Dummies* to be your second book
about caring for chickens. Your first chicken raising how-to
manual, *Raising Chickens For Dummies* by Kimberly Willis and Rob
Ludlow (John Wiley & Sons, Inc.), can help you begin with these
feathered friends by giving you plans for hen starter homes and
dropping hints about critical basic points on flock keeping, such
as, "hens don't need a rooster to lay eggs." That book touches on
chicken health problems, but *Chicken Health For Dummies* can take
you to the next level — what you *need* to know as a small flock
keeper about keeping chickens healthy and treating illnesses and
injuries. We wrote this book so that you can have an easy-to-use
reference for poultry preventive care and chicken repair.

We're confident that every procedure we guide you through is
doable and practical in a backyard setting — because we've used
the procedures ourselves to manage our own backyard flocks.

Another great part about this book is that you decide where to start and what to read. It's a reference you can jump into and out of at will. Just head to the table of contents or index to find the information you want.

Conventions Used in This Book

We use the following conventions throughout the text to make things consistent and easy to understand:

- ✔ All web addresses appear in `monofont`.

- ✔ New terms appear in *italics* and are closely followed by an easy-to-understand definition.

- ✔ **Bold** is used to highlight the action parts of numbered steps and emphasize keywords.

Traditionally, books about animal health refer to livestock in a gender-neutral way, but we feel coldhearted calling a hard-working, personable hen or rooster "it." The majority of backyard chickens are female, in part because rowdy roosters are unwelcome in many suburban and urban communities, so we bow to majority rule and refer to any chicken with the pronouns *she, her,* and *hers* (except when we are specifically talking about male chickens, in which case, *he, him,* and *his* apply). We also use the word *who,* not *that,* to refer to our poultry companions. *It* and *its* are reserved for chicks or birds of unknown gender and inanimate objects.

What You're Not to Read

Although we're attached to every word on these pages, and we hope you feel the same way, we understand if you don't read the book cover to cover, and want to skip around instead. That's why we've set some text off from the main information, stuff that will fascinate poultry science nerds and start some unusual conversations at parties, but it's not crucial for most small flock keepers to know. You can live without reading these items, but they're interesting, so come back to them when you get a moment. These items are:

- ✔ **Text in sidebars:** Sidebars are shaded boxes that discuss poultry science topics in more depth or give information that's important to a small segment of flock keepers, such as organic producers.

- ✔ **Anything with a Technical Stuff icon:** If the information in these tidbits applies to your exceptional situation, you'll be really glad we answered your pressing, but not-so-common technical question.

Foolish Assumptions

We love to talk chicken: broilers, gamefowl, bantams, wild jungle-fowl, and fowl of all purposes and all sizes — they're universally interesting to us. Going off on a tangent would be easy for us (What's your favorite "Why did the chicken cross the road" joke?), so to keep us focused on what you, a backyard flock keeper, want to know about chicken health, we need to understand your goals and concerns. We figure that your goals and concerns are similar to ours, because we're backyard flock keepers, too. Based on that connection, here's what we assume about you:

- ✔ Although you have some basic knowledge of chickens, you aren't a poultry expert.

- ✔ You take care of chickens (or plan to) and you want to find out more about keeping them healthy.

- ✔ You like animals and believe that taking good care of them involves understanding their needs and treating them with kindness.

- ✔ You keep (or are planning to keep) a small home flock. You don't intend to raise chickens on a commercial scale of 1,000 or more laying hens or broilers.

- ✔ You have some very basic first aid, gardening, carpentry, or crafts skills (or a friend who has these skills) and a desire to use them.

- ✔ You're not afraid to handle chickens or get your hands dirty.

Some things we *won't* assume about you are the reasons you keep chickens or your specific flock keeping philosophy. We think chickens are great, for many reasons — they're great for pets, eggs, meat, competition, a small family business, garden decorations, and more. In this book, we try to include a wide range of perspectives of small flock keeping. We're sure you can find tips and information in these pages that can suit your style of flock keeping, whatever that may be.

Just as you're certain to find advice in these pages that suits your particular style, you're bound to come across some uncomfortable notions, too. Is a diapered apartment chicken not your kind of pet? Skip that point and move on to the next. Does the thought of eating a chicken disturb you? Forgive us, please; the references to the nutritional qualities of chicken eggs or meat aren't aimed at you, but someone else who values that information.

How This Book Is Organized

Chicken Health For Dummies is organized into seven parts. We provide a nugget of an explanation for each part's topic here.

Part I: The Healthy Chicken

In order to spot a sick chicken, you need to know how a normal one looks and behaves. In Chapter 2, we provide a primer on chicken anatomy and body functions, so you can recognize a healthy chicken, inside and out. Chapter 3 gives a view of fowl society, behavior, and communication. Chapters 4, 5, and 6 focus on maintaining a healthy flock by keeping chickens clean, comfortable, and well-fed.

Part II: Recognizing Signs of Chicken Illness

How do you know a chicken is sick? In this part, we help you distinguish normal from abnormal chicken body functions and behavior, narrow down the possibilities to get you closer to a diagnosis, and provide advice about common concerns of flock keepers. We cover the most common ailments of adult chickens in Chapter 8 and health problems of chicks in Chapter 9. Chapter 10 tackles the extremes of chicken disease: mild, hard-to-put-your-finger-on-it illnesses on one end of the spectrum, and mysterious sudden death on the other.

Part III: A Close-Up Examination of Chicken Woes and Diseases

In this part, we discuss the major chicken diseases, briefing you on the cause, the signs and means of spread, prevention tips, and treatment advice. The chapters in this part are very helpful if you need to zoom in to a particular chicken disease that you've heard about. Wonder why you should buy chicks from a pullorum-clean flock? Chapter 12 is the place to look. Worried about worms? Check out Chapter 13.

Part IV: Your Chicken Repair Manual (and Advice for When to Close the Book)

We get down to the dirty work in this part. Here we help you make a diagnosis for a flock problem, whether you have the help of a chicken health advisor, or you're on your own. We show you how to do basic procedures, such as giving an injection or trimming a wing. Finally, we provide advice on closing the repair manual and killing a sick or injured chicken humanely.

Part V: The Chicken/Human Interface

The chicken/human interface is the time and place where chicken health and human health collide. These accidents can happen, but they're not common and they're rarely serious. What's good for you is often good for your chickens, and vice versa. Find ways to protect yourself and your chickens in this part.

Part VI: The Part of Tens

In this part, we take ten questions that we hear backyard flock keepers ask frequently and we answer them as succinctly as possible. We also take on ten common misconceptions about chicken health and present the facts, briefly.

Appendix

The appendix contains a few important lists. We're sure you'll find the chart of medication dosages for chickens in small flocks an extremely handy reference when you need it. The same goes for the list of disinfectants and the list of parasite treatments that we refer to in other parts of this book.

Icons Used in This Book

To make this book easier to read and simpler to use, we include some icons that can help you key in to main ideas.

This icon appears whenever an idea or item can save you time, money, or stress when taking care of your chickens.

Any time you see this icon, you know the information that follows is so important that it's worth reading more than once.

This icon flags information that highlights dangers to your chicken's well-being or to human health.

This icon appears next to information that's interesting, but isn't essential for all backyard flock keepers to know.

Where to Go from Here

Although starting at the beginning is customary, this book is organized so you can jump to whatever chapter you urgently need and find complete information. Got a sick hen? Head straight for Chapter 8. Concerned about a chick? Go to Chapter 9. Are you standing in the feed store, puzzling over crumbles or pellets? Check Chapter 6.

If you have no pressing concerns and all's well in the backyard, you may want to start with Part I, which can help you keep your happy flock healthy. You can also peruse the table of contents or index, find a topic that interests you, and go there. We wish you and your coop's residents health and good fortune!

Part I
The Healthy Chicken

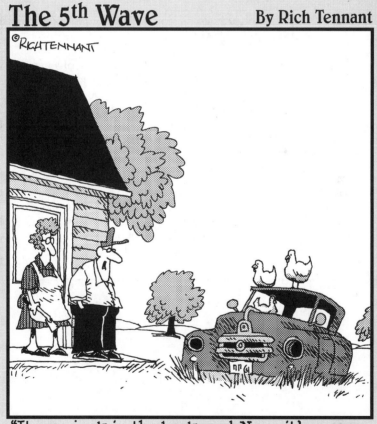

The 5th Wave   By Rich Tennant

"It <u>was</u> junk in the backyard. Now, it's a 1952 Nash chicken coupe."

In this part...

*1*n Part I, we give you a view — inside and out — of a hen and her family, and we tour the fascinating behavior of chickens in chicken society. Why do we wax poetic about healthy chickens in a book about chicken health problems? First, you can't recognize a sick chicken if you aren't thoroughly familiar with healthy ones. And second, attending to a chicken's behavioral needs (respecting her chickeness?) avoids many preventable stress-related illnesses and injuries.

The keys to chicken health are keeping the flock clean, comfortable, and well fed. We glean tips from wisdom handed down by generations of flock keepers to share with you in this part of the book.

Chapter 1

A Picture of Backyard Flock Health

*C*hickens have fascinated people for thousands of years, ever since humans and red junglefowl met in Southeast Asia and began a productive relationship together. Humans have taken full advantage of the partnership and of the chicken's versatility. The wild junglefowl hen lays a scanty 15 to 30 eggs a year; after thousands of years of selection and care by people, modern domesticated hens can surpass the 300-egg-per-year mark. Today, chicken meat is a major source of protein for human nutrition around the globe.

People clearly benefit from the human/chicken bond, but what does the chicken get out of this relationship? In exchange for eggs, meat, entertainment, and a wholesome connection with nature, backyard flock keepers protect their birds from danger and disease, and free them from worries of finding a good meal and a cozy place to sleep at night. In this book, we offer advice to help you keep up your end of the bargain.

Ideally, flock keepers also remember that chickens are, down deep, still wild junglefowl, driven to dustbathe, forage, and establish pecking orders. Caretakers can and should provide opportunities for chickens to be chickens and to express their inner junglefowl.

In this chapter, we introduce you to backyard chickens, their troubles, and what you can do to prevent health problems and respond to unfortunate events.

Introducing the Backyard Chicken

Throughout this book we make the distinction between backyard and commercial chicken flocks. Although you can probably point out general, sometimes overlapping differences between commercial and backyard flocks in terms of management style, reasons for raising chickens, types of birds, and farm sizes, we stick with a simple definition. For the purpose of this book, we consider a farm with 1,000 or more chickens a *commercial flock,* and call a place with fewer than 1,000 chickens a *backyard flock.*

Okay, 999 birds is *extreme* backyard flock keeping, and as you may suspect, most backyard flocks have far fewer than 1,000 birds. The majority of backyard flock keepers in the United States have fewer than 25 chickens, according to informal surveys.

You may already be savvy to the lingo of backyard flock keepers, but to keep us all on the same page, we provide a list of poultry terms used in this book:

- **Pullet/hen:** In poultry show circles, a pullet is a female chicken less than a year old, and a hen is a female chicken 1-year-old and up. Other folks consider a pullet to be a female chicken that has not yet laid an egg, and a hen as one who has.

- **Cockerel/rooster:** A cockerel is a male chicken less than a year old. A rooster is a male chicken 1-year-old and up.

- **Egg-type chickens:** Chickens of breeds developed for egg production. Commercial white egg layers are Leghorns, and commercial brown egg layers were developed from the Rhode Island Red, New Hampshire, and Plymouth Rock breeds of chicken.

- **Broiler:** A young chicken suitable for grilling, roasting, or barbecuing. Very fast-growing *meat-type* chickens that make excellent broilers were created from the Cornish and Plymouth Rock breeds of chickens. You may hear meat-type chickens described as "Cornish cross" or "Cornish Rocks."

- **Dual-purpose chickens:** Chickens of breeds that are suitable for both egg and meat production, such as the Delaware or Plymouth Rock breeds.

- **Gamefowl:** Chickens of breeds developed for the purpose of producing fighting cocks, such as the Modern Game and the Old English Game breeds.

- **Bantams:** Very small chickens belonging to breeds that are often miniature versions of larger chicken breeds.

Backyard menageries are the norm

In a 2004 USDA survey, backyard flock keepers were asked what types of birds they kept. Four out of five flocks had more than one type of bird. The following shows the percentage of backyard flocks that had different types of chickens and other birds:

Chickens

- ✔ Chickens for egg production: 63 percent

- ✔ Gamefowl: 23 percent

- ✔ Chickens for meat production: 17 percent

- ✔ Show chickens: 10 percent

Other types of birds

- ✔ Ducks: 21 percent

- ✔ Guinea fowl: 12 percent

- ✔ Turkeys: 7 percent

- ✔ Caged pet birds: 4 percent

The 2004 USDA backyard chicken study is the most recent scientific survey on this topic. You can read the entire report to get a bigger picture of U.S. backyard flocks at www.aphis. usda.gov/animal_health/ nahms/poultry/downloads/ poultry04/Poultry04_dr_ PartI.pdf.

> ✔ **Heritage breed chickens:** Chickens belonging to breeds that were recognized by the American Poultry Association prior to the mid–20th century. Heritage chickens are ideal for backyard settings, because they're active, long-lived, outdoor foragers.

 Visit the American Livestock Breeds Conservancy website at www. albc-usa.org/heritagechicken/definition.html for more information about heritage breed chickens.

Creating a Healthy and Contented Life for Your Flock

A free-range backyard hen seems to have an idyllic life, enjoying the freedom to scratch and forage for interesting, wiggly things to eat, and experiencing the contentment that comes with flopping in a dustbath and snuggling close with her flock mates on a night-time perch. See Chapter 3 for a more complete account of chicken behaviors that apparently express a cheerful enjoyment of life.

A backyard hen, however, trades that full and interesting life for a higher risk of early death due to predators or disease, compared to hens kept in cages on commercial poultry farms. In fact, surveys from around the world have shown that the typical mortality rate in free-range chicken flocks is at least twice the mortality rate of flocks kept in cages.

Despite the stacked odds, you can prevent many of the injuries and illnesses in backyard chickens. That's why good management of a backyard flock is so important — to make sure that rich quality of life is also a long and healthy life. These sections highlight a few areas that you can help make your flock safer and sound. Chapters 4, 5, and 6 cover additional ways to protect your flock by keeping your birds clean, comfortable, and well fed.

Recognizing risky free-range encounters

Almost all backyard flocks are *free-range* — by that, we mean they have at least part-time access to the outdoors. Some backyard flock keepers have an extremely liberal free-range policy and allow their chickens to roam away from their backyards; the rest confine their birds to a yard, coop, barn, or less commonly, cages.

Most backyard flocks have regular contact with other animals. The animals that often coexist in a backyard with a flock keeper's chickens are

---

Meeting your fellow flock keepers

You probably have a lot in common with other backyard flock keepers, including your reasons for keeping chickens, where you get them, and how you care for them. If you're just getting started with raising chickens, you're in a large class of students; our informal poll suggests to us that most U.S. backyard flock keepers have been raising birds for less than three years.

By far, having fresh eggs is the most important and common reason that people keep backyard chickens. When we ask backyard flock keepers why they keep poultry, they often tell us the following reasons, listed roughly in order of importance:

- Eating fresh eggs
- Having chickens as pets
- Controlling bugs with a foraging flock
- Fertilizing a garden with chicken manure
- Eating fresh meat
- Exhibiting at poultry shows
- Making extra income from selling eggs, meat, or birds

- Wild birds

- Flock keeper's dogs or cats

- Neighbors' dogs or cats

- Neighbors' poultry

Free-range chickens risk becoming the neighborhood dogs' next snack (or chew toy), or picking up an infectious disease from wild birds or someone else's backyard poultry. See Chapter 4 for tips on protecting your flock from hazards outside of your yard with common sense biosecurity measures.

Feeding chickens for good health and production

Feed is the major ongoing expense of raising chickens. Good nutrition pays off in healthy chickens who lay lots of eggs, so wise flock keepers carefully consider what they pour into the feeder each day. Chickens must get protein, energy, vitamins, and minerals from their food. Daily requirements for these nutrients change according to the bird's age and occupation. Flock keepers can choose among different diet formulas for different types of chickens and stages of life, including:

- **Meat-type chicken starter, grower, and finisher diets:** These rations are intended for broiler chicks as they grow up.

- **Egg-type or dual-purpose chicken starter, grower, and finisher diets:** These rations are designed for feeding chicks destined to lay eggs. They work well for young pet chickens.

- **Layer diets:** These rations are formulated for hens laying eggs for eating or hatching.

Commercially prepared feed takes the guesswork out of chicken nutrition. The tag on the feed bag tells you what type of chicken the feed is designed for, and how to feed it. Flock keepers can prepare nutritious homemade chicken feed, but that's a project that takes more time, skill, and attention to detail than opening a bag of complete commercial chicken feed. Chapter 6 provides more information about practical options for feeding your flock well.

What Can Go Wrong?

Chickens that are well fed and kept in clean, comfortable quarters have remarkable natural resistance to disease. As tough and resilient as chickens are, however, they're far from invulnerable or immortal.

Despite your best care, you're likely to be faced with a sick chicken at some point in your flock-keeping career. In this book, we cover common health problems of adult chickens and chicks, guide you to a diagnosis for puzzling signs of illness, and help you investigate sudden death when it occurs in your flock. Read on for a preview.

Common health problems

In general, larger backyard flocks are more likely to suffer health problems than smaller flocks. Closed flocks (ones in which no new birds are introduced) are less likely to catch something than flocks where birds come and go. The following list gives common backyard chicken health problems along with the chapters in this book where you can find more information:

✔ External parasites, such as mites, lice, and fleas (see Chapter 13)

✔ Unexplained death (see Chapter 10)

✔ Respiratory signs, such as cough, sneeze, swollen face, or discharge from nostrils or eyes (check out Chapters 8 and 9)

✔ Weight loss (refer to Chapter 10)

✔ Diarrhea (check out Chapters 8 and 9)

✔ Droopy birds (birds who show they don't feel well for any number of reasons by drooping their heads) (see Chapter 10)

✔ Lameness (refer to Chapters 8 and 9)

✔ Decreased egg production (check out Chapter 10)

✔ Neurologic signs, such as lack of coordination and weakness (flip to Chapters 8 and 9)

Major causes of death

Most backyard flock keepers experience the death of at least one of their chickens each year (other than chickens slaughtered for human consumption). On average, about one out of ten chickens in a backyard flock dies during one year (a mortality rate of about 10 percent).

The following list shows major causes of death for free-range hens that we compiled from a number of surveys around the world. We list them roughly in order of importance along with the chapter where we discuss the cause of death in greater detail.

✔ **Predator attacks:** Almost everywhere in North America, raccoons, opossums, foxes, and skunks prowl around chicken coops, and hawks and owls patrol the skies. These predators love a nice chicken dinner. See Chapter 11 for how to protect your flock from four-legged and winged marauders.

- ✔ **Cannibalism or vent pecking:** They're aggressive acts by flock mates; refer to Chapter 11.

- ✔ **Colibacillosis:** Also called egg peritonitis; check out Chapter 12.

- ✔ **Vent prolapse:** This is when part of the internal reproductive tract becomes misplaced and protrudes outside a hen's body; refer to Chapter 8.

- ✔ **Fatty liver hemorrhagic syndrome:** This is internal bleeding from a diseased liver; see Chapter 10.

 Flock keepers can take many precautions to prevent predator attacks, cannibalism, and vent pecking, three of the most common causes of death for backyard hens.

Doing Your Part to Keep Your Flock Fit

Preventing disease is far more successful and less frustrating for small flock keepers than treating health problems after they appear in the flock. We emphasize prevention over cure throughout this book.

Although you can't keep your chickens in a sterile bubble, we have some practical tips to help you maintain a healthy flock. Start your flock with disease-free chickens, and help keep them that way by choosing new birds wisely and building biosecurity routines into daily flock chores.

All's not lost if a minor disease does show up in your flock. Often, you can medicate or vaccinate chickens to limit the damage, and chicken health advisors are available to coach you in your battle against flock ailments.

Safely sourcing new birds

About one-third of backyard flock keepers in the United States introduce at least one new bird each year to the flock. Most flock keepers get their birds from friends or neighbors, a feed store, or by mail-order. Auctions, flea markets, fairs, and shows are other places where chickens destined for backyards can be found. Bringing home new birds is risky business, because a flock keeper can unknowingly bring home an infectious disease along with a new chicken.

 Some sources and age groups of chickens are riskier to bring home than others. Generally, younger chickens are less likely to be carriers of infectious diseases than older ones, so hatching eggs and day-old chicks are safer to add to a flock than adult birds. (Notice we didn't say "completely safe.") See Chapter 4 for more tips on reducing risk to your flock when you introduce new birds.

Practicing biosecurity

Biosecurity is a set of practices — things you do every day — that helps keep infectious organisms, such as viruses and bacteria, out of your flock. If a disease-causing organism manages to find its way into your flock, the same biosecurity practices can help prevent the spread of the disease between your chickens, or the spread outside your flock to someone else's chickens.

The following list presents some biosecurity practices that are practical for most backyard flock keepers:

- ✔ Control rodents in bird areas
- ✔ Isolate new birds before adding them to an existing flock
- ✔ Keep birds confined to their own yard
- ✔ Change clothes between visiting other birds and caring for own flock
- ✔ Dedicate footwear for bird area or clean footwear before entering bird area
- ✔ Wash hands before handling poultry

How does your biosecurity compare with that of your fellow flock keepers? Take the biosecurity self-assessment test in Chapter 4 to rate your efforts to protect your flock from infectious diseases.

Medicating and vaccinating backyard flocks

Flock keepers in the United States can purchase medications over the counter to treat their chickens according to the directions on the label. The most common place to buy them is at a local feed store. Backyard flock keepers most frequently use antibiotics, coccidiosis preventives or treatments, vitamins, and dewormers.

Any use of a medication in a way that isn't listed on the label is called *extra-label use,* which is illegal in the United States without a prescription from a licensed veterinarian. Talk to a veterinarian if you're considering using a medication for a chicken in an extra-label way.

Most backyard flock keepers don't find it necessary to vaccinate their chickens. We tend to agree, but we think vaccination may be useful in these circumstances:

- ✔ You take chickens to poultry shows and bring them back home.

- ✔ You buy chickens from auctions, poultry shows, or other places where birds gather, and add them to your existing flock.

- ✔ Your flock has had a vaccine-preventable disease problem in the past.

- ✔ Outbreaks of a vaccine-preventable chicken disease occur in the area where you live.

In Chapter 16, we show you how to administer medications and vaccinations to your chickens. The most common methods for getting medications or vaccinations into a chicken are by mouth, by eyedrop, into the skin of the wing web, or by injection under the skin or into a muscle.

Finding help for chicken health problems

Backyard flock keepers consult a variety of sources for chicken health advice, most often the Internet, feed store staff, or other flock keepers. A few flock keepers consult a veterinarian who is willing to work with poultry. We suggest the following go-to people who are in the best position to give you expert advice for treating a sick chicken or managing a backyard flock:

- ✔ Avian veterinarians

- ✔ Cooperative Extension Service agents

- ✔ Veterinary diagnostic laboratories

- ✔ Poultry nutritionists

- ✔ National Poultry Improvement Plan inspectors

- ✔ Poultry veterinarians

- ✔ State veterinarians

Chapter 15 offers suggestions for finding and working with these chicken-savvy professionals.

Disappearing poultry science departments

Quick! Take advantage of these sources of chicken-raising wisdom, before they're gone from your area. Poultry scientists investigate the best ways to manage flocks, hatch eggs, feed birds, and keep chickens healthy, so their knowledge and innovations are invaluable for flock keepers of all types and flock sizes.

Unfortunately, for several reasons, the number of poultry science departments at U.S. universities has declined by more than 80 percent in the last 50 years. The amount of poultry health research and the number of poultry researchers have also decreased with the shrinking departments. Because extension offices are closely tied to universities, the number of poultry experts that extension agents can tap into has decreased as well.

The following six poultry science departments were still standing at the time we wrote this book:

- Auburn University Department of Poultry Science (www.ag.auburn.edu/poul/)

- University of Arkansas Department of Poultry Science (www.poultryscience.uark.edu/)

- University of Georgia Department of Poultry Science (www.poultry.uga.edu)

- Mississippi State University Department of Poultry Science (www.poultry.msstate.edu)

- North Carolina State University Department of Poultry Science (www.cals.ncsu.edu/poultry/index.php)

- Texas A&M University Poultry Science Department (http://gallus.tamu.edu/)

Chapter 2

The Anatomy and Body Functions of the Happy, Healthy Chicken

*L*acking the ability to fly ourselves (or at least become momentarily airborne, chicken-style), we think the structure and function of birds' bodies is amazing. Curiosity is reason enough to figure out a bird's anatomy, but for flock keepers, some knowledge of the parts of a chicken and how they work is practical, too. If you know what's normal, you can recognize what's abnormal, and do something to fix the problem. You can also accurately describe the problem and communicate clearly with your chicken health advisor.

In this chapter, we introduce you to the body systems of the chicken, which seem vaguely familiar to a mammal, but with some unique bird twists. The hen's egg-laying machinery is a topic of extreme interest for flock keepers, so we give some details on how the hen's edible "gifts" are delivered several times a week. Finally, we describe a chick developing within the egg, hatching, and growing up to become a personable, useful member of a backyard flock.

Taking a Closer Look at Chicken Parts: The Body Systems

Chickens and other birds have a number of specialized features — characteristics that make them unique in the animal kingdom. Most of the specializations are related to getting off the ground and into the air. Here are a few of the most remarkable body features:

- **Feathers:** Feathers conserve heat and streamline the body. A feather is amazingly strong for something so light and flexible.

- **A light-weight skeleton:** Aircraft designers must wish they could use those super-light bird bones as construction materials.

- **Simple digestive and urinary systems:** No teeth, short intestines, and no bladder are also weight-saving features.

- **Reproductive organs:** They shrink when they're not being used.

We hope we've sparked your curiosity about the fascinating body systems of chickens. In the next sections, we give you more highlights of chicken anatomy and physiology.

The outside of the chicken: Eyes, ears, skin, and feathers

Being able to refer to the common names of the outside parts of the chicken is helpful when describing a problem to someone long distance. Refer to Figure 2-1 as you read the following list and see the outside parts of a chicken:

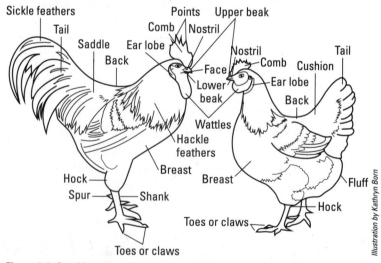

Figure 2-1: Outside parts of a rooster and a hen.

✔ **Eyes:** Chickens have better vision than people, by several measures. Their ability to bring objects into sharp focus and to notice very small differences in color is better than human vision, even in newly hatched chicks. Chickens can even see ultraviolet light. (Unless you have super-human powers, you can't.) In case you were wondering, the most common chicken eye color is reddish-brown.

A chicken's upper and lower eyelids aren't meant for blinking. Instead, chickens have a third eyelid for that — the thin, translucent *nictitating membrane*. When it's not in use, the third eyelid is stowed in the corner of the eye nearest the beak. It acts like a windshield wiper, or sometimes, safety goggles. A chicken reflexively pulls the third eyelid up over the eye whenever she needs to clear some eye gunk or avoid flying debris (or a kid's curious finger). When a chicken is sleeping, the lower lid is pulled up to close the eye; the upper eyelid doesn't move much.

✔ **Ears:** A fringe of feathers surrounds the opening to a chicken's ears. This opening leads to a canal that ends at the ear drum. Chickens' sensitivity to sound and ability to hear low and high pitched sounds is similar to human hearing ability.

✔ **Skin:** The skin of chickens is very thin and stretchy compared to yours. Chicken skin has no sweat glands. You can find skin glands on a chicken's body in only two places:

- **The ear canal:** The glands in chicken's ear canals have the same function yours do: making ear wax, which provides a barrier to germs and water.

- **The base of the tail:** The *preen* gland, also called the *uropygial* (say it: yur-o-*pie*-jee-el) gland or *oil gland,* is on the back of the chicken where the tail meets the body. It produces oily stuff that a chicken works into her plumage with her beak. We suspect she does this to make her feathers water resistant, but there may be other beauty secrets involving preen gland oil that she's not sharing with us.

✔ **Feathers:** Chickens have between 7,500 and 9,000 feathers (someone counted them!), that are made of the protein *keratin,* the same stuff that beaks, horns, hooves, hair, and fingernails are made of. Chickens shed old worn-out feathers and replace them with new ones in a normal, orderly process of *molting.* Molt is an annual event for most chickens, typically happening in the fall, although stress or changes in weather can trigger molting, too. Molt follows a regular pattern of feather loss over areas of the body, in this order: head, neck, breast, body, wings, and finally, tail. Large wing feathers are dropped in a definite order, starting at the center of the wing and working out toward the wing tip and then, from the center of the wing toward the body. The process of molting can take as little as six weeks, or as long as six months, depending on the bird.

How a hen molts can give you a clue about her egg-laying prowess. Your best layers are the ones who quickly finish molting, and they often look terrible while it's happening — they're the raggedy hens with bald patches. The pretty girls who molt gradually and never have "bad plumage days" probably don't produce many eggs.

✔ **Toes:** Chickens have four or five toes, depending on the breed. Bony outgrowths on the insides of the legs, called *spurs,* appear in both males and females, although spurs are more well-developed on roosters.

✔ **Combs and wattles:** The *comb* is a fleshy crest on top of a chicken's head. *Wattles* are the pair of skin flaps hanging from a chicken's throat. Both males and females have combs and wattles, which come in a variety of sizes and shapes, also depending on the breed of the chicken.

Breathing and circulating blood

The main job of the respiratory system of birds is to absorb oxygen and rid the body of carbon dioxide. In addition, the respiratory system also gets rid of excess heat, detoxifies some of the waste products of the body, and makes noise — most noticeably, crowing noise, much to the annoyance of our neighbors.

Like humans, birds have a windpipe and two lungs, but from there, birds are distinctly unlike mammals. Air flows into a bird's lungs during the intake of breath, it continues through the lungs into nine *air sacs,* and then it goes back out through the lungs again. Birds get two doses of oxygen for the price of one breath! The air sacs are arranged around the inside of the chest and abdominal cavity, and they connect with some of the bones of the skeleton, as Figure 2-2 shows.

Humans breathe with the help of the diaphragm muscle, which divides the chest and abdominal cavities. Birds don't have a working diaphragm; instead, a bird moves its rib cage and *keel* (breastbone) to draw air into the lungs and force it back out.

Holding a chick or other small bird firmly around the body stops them from breathing, and it may quickly kill them. This is just one of several reasons why small children should be supervised when holding chicks.

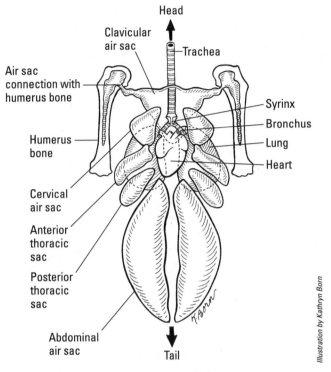

Figure 2-2: The respiratory system of a chicken.

The voice box in chickens is called the *syrinx,* located down in the chest cavity where the windpipe splits to enter each lung. Both male and female chickens have a syrinx, so hens can crow, too, if they feel like it. The syrinx isn't an optional piece of anatomy though. A rooster can't live with his syrinx removed. We talk more about chickens' voices in Chapter 3.

The layout of a chicken's heart isn't so different from the layout of a human heart. It has four chambers and pumps blood through two loops: one loop through the lungs, and the other loop through the rest of the body. A bird's heart is relatively large for its body size, compared to mammal hearts.

Eating and digestion

Having a firm understanding of a chicken's digestion system can help you figure out the reason behind a chicken's digestive upsets. Figure 2-3 shows the layout of the chicken digestive system, beginning to end. Refer to this figure as we explain the different parts in the following list:

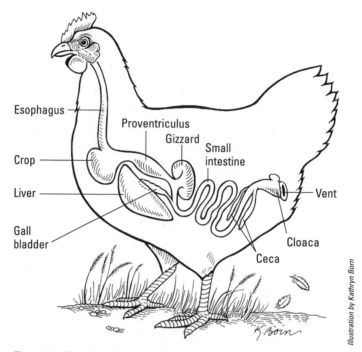

Illustration by Kathryn Born

Figure 2-3: The digestive system of a chicken.

- ✔ **Mouth:** A chicken can't physically stick out her tongue or say "Ahh," so you may never see the inside of a chicken's mouth. If you have, you probably noticed the gaping hole in the roof of the mouth that connects with the nasal passages. What you saw wasn't a defect. The gap is known in chicken anatomy circles as the *choana,* and it closes when a chicken swallows, so the bird can't do the "milk coming out of the nose" trick.

- ✔ **Crop:** Chickens don't have teeth, so they can't chew food in their mouths. A chicken picks up food in her beak and swallows it with the help of her tongue. The food travels down the esophagus to the *crop* (which is really just a bulge in the esophagus), where the chicken stores the food until she can digest it at her leisure.

- ✔ **Esophagus, stomach, and gizzard:** The esophagus continues past the crop to the true stomach, the *proventriculus,* where digestion really gets rolling with the addition of hydrochloric acid and digestive enzymes. The food still hasn't been chewed, though. That happens a little farther down the line in the *gizzard* (also known as the *ventriculus*), which is another unique anatomical feature of birds. This muscular organ acts as the bird's teeth to grind the food and mix it with digestive juices, with the help of several small stones that have been hanging out inside the gizzard, ever since the chicken ate them a while back.

If a chicken eats a small sharp object, like a staple or a bit of wire, it's likely to get stuck in the gizzard. With all the grinding going on, the sharp object can eventually wear a hole through the gizzard, slowly killing the chicken. Be careful to keep your coop and yard free of small, sharp metal objects, or broken glass.

✔ **Digestive tract:** Chickens have a pancreas, liver, and intestines, which pretty much do the same things as they do in humans. The digestive tract layout differs, though, when you get to the *cecum.* The plural of cecum is *ceca,* which is useful to know, because birds have two. The ceca are blind pouches located where the small and large intestines come together. Birds extract a little extra nutrition out of their meal, especially fatty acids and B vitamins, through the fermentation process that happens in the ceca.

The ceca empty their contents a couple of times a day, producing nasty-smelling, pasty droppings. Chicken owners should be familiar with these normal but smelly "cecal poops."

✔ **Kidneys and vent:** Chickens don't pee, and they don't have a bladder. Urinary system wastes (*urates* is the word used for bird urine) produced by the kidneys are simply dumped in with the digestive wastes at the end of the digestive system, at the *cloaca,* or *vent.* That's why normal chicken droppings contain white urates mixed with darker digested material.

Moving around: The skeletal system

Besides the obvious role of holding up the chicken, the skeletal system has at least two additional important functions: calcium storage, and believe it or not, breathing! See Figure 2-4 for an illustration of the skeleton of the chicken.

Two types of bones make up the bird skeletal system:

✔ **Pneumatic:** These bones (say it: new-*matic*) are hollow and connected to the respiratory system via the air sacs. Examples of pneumatic bones are the skull, collar bone (clavicle), pelvis, and bones of the lower back.

✔ **Medullary:** These bones, including the leg bones, ribs, and shoulder blades, serve as a source of stored calcium for the hen to tap into to make strong egg shells. Bone marrow filling the centers of the medullary bones makes red and white blood cells.

A number of beefed-up features to the bones support the wings and allow flight. The backbones in the chest cavity are fused together, and the ribs overlap, making an extremely strong and rigid rib cage. The keel provides a large surface area for the wing muscles to attach.

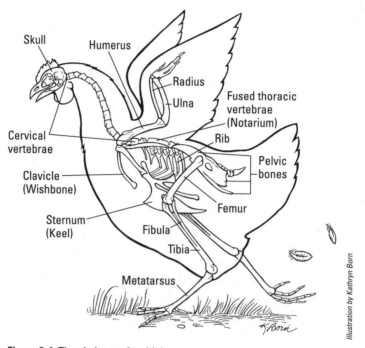

Illustration by Kathryn Born

Figure 2-4: The skeleton of a chicken.

Although the chicken's skeleton implies good flying skills, a chicken's muscles tell a different story — chickens are better walkers than flyers. Chicken breast meat is white, because the majority of muscle cells there are the type cut out for short bursts of activity, not long flights. The main type of muscle cells in the dark meat of legs and thighs are meant for sustained effort, such as walking around. Other types of birds that are better flyers than chickens have all dark meat muscle.

Defending against disease

We give you a run-down of the chicken immune system, to familiarize you with that defense network, because flock owners need to know how to help their chickens protect themselves against and deal with infectious diseases. A bird has built-in defenses against invading disease-causing organisms, such as bacteria or viruses. Figure 2-5 shows the parts of a chicken's defense network. The following list walks you through these different parts of a chicken's immune system:

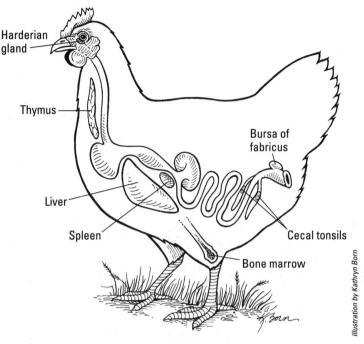

Harderian gland

Thymus

Bursa of fabricus

Liver

Spleen

Cecal tonsils

Bone marrow

Illustration by Kathryn Born

Figure 2-5: The organs of a chicken's immune system.

✔ **General:** Some of the immune defenses are general, which means that they guard against a wide range of organisms, rather than a specific one. Unbroken skin is the frontline of the general defense network against disease. The microbes that normally live on the skin and in the gut also defend against invasion attempts by foreign organisms. The lining of a chicken's windpipe, like that of other animals, is covered with mucous and waving hairs, called *cilia,* that collect and sweep inhaled dust and other gunk (like bacteria) up and away from the lungs. Maybe the sweltering body temperature of chickens, which fluctuates a couple of degrees around 106 degrees Fahrenheit (41 degrees Celsius) in healthy chickens, discourages some types of disease-causing organisms from setting up shop. Also, genes play a role in protecting some strains of chickens against some illnesses.

✔ **Antibodies:** Like humans and other animals, chickens make *antibodies,* which are very specific defense molecules programmed against particular organisms. For example, antibodies for infectious bronchitis virus protect chickens only against infectious bronchitis virus, and not Newcastle disease virus (for more on those diseases, see Chapter 12). A chick can receive antibodies from a mother hen through the egg. These hen-donated antibodies last for the first couple of weeks of the chick's life, protecting the chick until her immune system is up and running, producing antibodies of her own.

In mammals, the spleen, tonsils, bone marrow, lymph nodes, and the *thymus* (a spongy thingy in the upper chest of young animals) are organs that have important roles in making antibodies and other molecules of the immune defense network. Birds have all that, too, except for the lymph nodes, and birds keep their tonsils in their ceca. Also, birds have a couple of other important outposts in the immune defense system: the *bursa of Fabricius,* which is a pouch above the cloaca of a young bird, and the *Harderian glands,* near each of the chicken's eyeballs.

Starting with the Chicken and then the Egg: Growth and Development

So what is the answer to the age-old question: Which came first, the chicken or the egg? Well, we don't know the answer, but in these sections, we start with the chicken and end up with a hatching egg. Along the way, we explain the reproductive ins and outs of chickens.

Reaching sexual maturity

Young female chickens *(pullets)* of modern breeds, such as commercial strains of Leghorns, start laying eggs at around 18 to 21 weeks of age and are 8 months old when they reach peak egg production. Old-fashioned or *heritage* breeds of chickens are late bloomers; they start laying eggs around 6 months of age. After a pullet reaches maturity, three things come together to determine when exactly she will lay her first egg:

- ✔ The number of hours of light she sees in a day
- ✔ Her weight
- ✔ Her body fat percentage

For a hen to lay eggs, a rooster's presence isn't necessary. For a hen to lay fertile, hatchable eggs, however, a rooster and his healthy reproductive system are vital necessities.

Starting at about 4 to 5 months of age, young roosters *(cockerels)* reach sexual maturity, producing sperm and acting like roosters. They can remain fertile for several years, although the quantity and quality of sperm that roosters produce decreases as they age.

During molt, and during the period of decreasing daylight hours in fall and winter, a hen usually takes a break and stops laying eggs. Her reproductive tract shrinks back to the size it was when she was a pullet. The rooster, too, takes a break in the short days of winter, and his fertility decreases for the season, to return in the spring.

Making eggs (and chicks, maybe)

In this section we discuss the birds and the bees, focusing on the birds, specifically reproduction by hens and roosters.

Reproducing from a hen's perspective

A female chick is hatched with a pair of ovaries and oviducts (left and right) and all the eggs she'll ever lay. After hatching though, only her left ovary and oviduct develops. If something goes wrong with the left ovary and oviduct during her life, she doesn't have a good backup plan.

When a hen is making eggs, or *in lay,* her ovary looks like a bunch of bright yellow grapes of various sizes. The egg-making process starts when one of the larger grapes is released from the ovary *(ovulation)* about 30 minutes after the previous egg is laid, usually in the morning, and almost never after 3 p.m.

Figure 2-6 shows the reproductive and urinary systems of the hen.

The big yellow grape released from the ovary will be the yolk of a new egg. The first part of the oviduct, the *infundibulum,* looks and acts like a catcher's mitt to catch the released yolk. If a rooster's sperm fertilizes the egg, it happens in the infundibulum. From there, the developing egg travels through the rest of the two-foot-long oviduct. In order, the sections of the oviduct are the magnum, isthmus, shell gland, and vagina, which ends at the cloaca from which the egg is laid. Table 2-1 shows the timeline and the event occurring at each stop in the route through the hen's oviduct. The total assembly line takes about 25 to 26 hours.

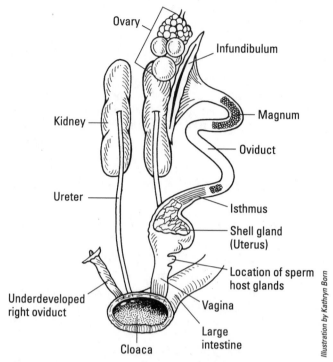

Figure 2-6: A hen's urinary and reproductive systems.

Illustration by Kathryn Born

Table 2-1	The Egg Assembly Line	
Station	*Time at Station*	*What Part Is Added*
Infundibulum	15 minutes	Yolk, sperm (if it's a fertilized model)
Magnum	3 hours	Egg white
Isthmus	75 minutes	Shell membranes
Shell gland	20 hours	Shell (obviously), eggshell pigment (optional)
Vagina	Not long (a few seconds)	Bloom, also called the *cuticle* (a waxy protective coating)

Eyeing the rooster's role in reproduction

A rooster keeps all his reproductive equipment inside. His pair of bean-shaped testicles is tucked up inside the abdomen, along the backbone, just above the kidneys. Male birds differ from their mammal counterparts in another important way — a rooster's sperm stays fresh at normal (hot!) chicken body temperature, while male mammals must keep their sperm slightly cooler than body temperature in external testicles.

From each of the rooster's testicles, a tube called the *ductus def-erens* carries sperm to the cloaca (see Figure 2-7). The rooster doesn't seem to miss having a functional copulatory organ, and mating is accomplished simply by placing his cloaca next to the hen's cloaca, and depositing sperm there.

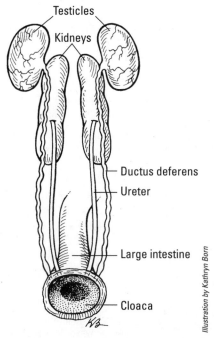

Testicles

Kidneys

Ductus deferens

Ureter

Large intestine

Cloaca

Illustration by Kathryn Born

Figure 2-7: A rooster's reproductive and urinary systems.

What happens after the deed is done

After mating, the hen stores the sperm in the tiny *sperm host glands,* located between the vagina and the shell gland of the oviduct. The sperm can live in the sperm host glands for about two weeks after mating. When an egg is laid, some sperm are squeezed out of the glands and they migrate up the oviduct to fertilize the next egg in the pipeline. This is a good backup plan, because if something happens to the man of the flock, the hens can still lay fertile eggs for a while after he's gone.

Hens will lay fertile eggs as soon as the second day after a sexually active and fertile rooster is introduced to the flock. It may take him a few days to make the rounds and mate with all the hens, so give him a week before expecting to see a high level of fertility in the eggs.

The mystery of sex determination in chickens

The sex of an individual animal is usually determined by genes on one of two sex chromosomes. Normally, each individual gets one sex chromosome from each parent. In people (and other mammals), sex chromosomes are labeled X and Y. Boys have one of each type of chromosome (XY) while girls have two X chromosomes (XX). The Y chromosome, contributed by the father, determines maleness.

Birds, as we point out repeatedly, seem to follow completely different sets of biological rules, from a mammal's perspective. Acknowledging that "dare to be different" approach, biologists label birds' two sex chromosomes Z and W. The Z chromosome, like mammals' X chromosome, is much bigger than the stubby W or Y chromosome. That's where the similarities end, however. Hens have one of each of the two types of chromosomes (ZW), and roosters have two copies of Z (ZZ). So it's the hen, by giving either a Z or W chromosome to each chick, who determines the sex of her offspring, instead of the father.

The Z and W sex chromosomes are involved in sex-linked colorations of some chickens, which allow you to identify the sex of chicks at hatch by obvious color differences in their downy feathers. A sex-linked gene, such as the gene that causes dark stripes *(barring)* on feathers, is found on the Z chromosome, which a female chick will never inherit from her mother.

The puzzling thing is that biologists don't know whether it's the W or the Z chromosome that matters most in determining sex in chickens. Does the W chromosome cause femaleness, or is it the double-dose of Z that makes a chicken male? That remains a mystery, but recent research suggests the answer is — both! Maybe there is no winner in the battle of the (chicken) sexes.

Knowing what goes on in the egg

A chicken egg is a complete package of nutrition and protection for the developing embryo chick. The yolk, egg white, and shell provide all the nutrients the embryo needs for the 21-day incubation period.

The embryo develops from the *ovum,* a small white dot on the surface of the yolk, which contains half the genes of a new chick. The other half of the new chick's genes comes from one of a rooster's sperm cells, which fertilized the ovum inside the hen's oviduct.

By the time the egg is laid the day after fertilization, the embryo has already been busy, dividing from that single-cell ovum into a blob of several thousand cells (although the embryo is still too small for you to see without a microscope). After the egg emerges from the nice warm hen into a cold world (below 68 degrees F/20 degrees C), the embryo stops developing, unless the egg is rewarmed by a sitting hen or an artificial incubator.

The ideal incubation temperature for chicken eggs is 99–100 degrees F (37–38 degrees C). At room temperature (actually, between 68 degrees F [13 degrees C] and ideal incubation temperature), the embryo can start to develop, but probably won't survive to hatch. The best temperature range for storing hatching eggs is between 55–68 degrees F (13–20 degrees C); the embryo is in suspended animation at those temperatures.

During incubation, the healthy embryo develops in a predictable way. We list the developmental milestones of a developing chicken embryo in Table 2-2.

Table 2-2	What to Expect When You're Incubating
Stage of Incubation	*Developmental Milestone*
Day 0	Sperm fertilizes ovum in the oviduct of the hen.
Days 1–3	Development begins for head, eyes, ears, and backbone; heart begins to beat.
Days 4–6	Development begins for eye pigmentation, reproductive organs, and beak.
Days 7–9	Development begins for feathers and toes.
Day 12	Down feathers are visible.

(continued)

Table 2-2 *(continued)*	
Stage of Incubation	*Developmental Milestone*
Day 17	Chick tucks her head under her right wing.
Day 19	The yolk sac is drawn in to the abdomen.
Day 20	Chick chips a hole *(pips)* through the shell.
Day 21	Chick hatches.

Life Outside the Egg: A Chick's First Few Weeks

For the first few days after hatching, a chick can't maintain her own body temperature and needs to be kept warm, either by mother hen's body heat or by a supplemental heat source that you can provide. The egg yolk, which the chick absorbed into her abdomen during the last few days before hatching, provides an energy source to keep the chick going for a couple of days, while she's figuring out how to eat and drink.

Hatcheries can ship day-old chicks without food or water because a chick's absorbed yolk sac provides nutrients for a couple of days after hatching. Chicks get a faster, less risky start on life, however, if you can get them to eat and drink as soon as they're able.

Newly hatched chicks certainly aren't completely helpless like some animal babies. Chicks hatch with their eyes open, wearing a birthday suit of cozy down feathers, and are ready to move. However, their digestive tracts, immune systems, skin, and feathers still have a lot of growing to do in the first six weeks of life.

Enjoy your fluffy chicks while you can, because they soon will lose their fluff. The down-covered chick will change her feathers three more times before she grows up. Down is replaced by the first full set of feathers between 1 to 5 weeks of age. A partial molt happens between 7 to 9 weeks old, and an adolescent chicken's full set of feathers start coming in at about 13 weeks of age.

A growth spurt occurs in the chick between 7 to 12 weeks of age. At the end of that growth spurt, the young bird will be nearly the size of a mature bird and about three-quarters of her eventual grown-up weight. Several weeks later, the chick's adolescent pullet sisters are going through a second growth spurt, rapidly filling out their frames and putting on weight in the two weeks leading up to laying their first eggs.

Chapter 3

That's What Chickens Do: Healthy Chicken Behavior

● ●

In This Chapter

▶ Understanding your chickens, creatures of habit

▶ Finding food and avoiding predators are always on the fowl mind

▶ Discovering words Dr. Dolittle knows

▶ Watching waltzing and tidbitting roosters impress their hens

● ●

*Y*our chicken is talking to you. Are you listening? Squawks, clucks, cackles, and fowl growls all have specific meanings for chickens. People have translated dozens of these vocalizations. Beyond the obvious noise associated with activities of daily living, chickens also communicate through body language, which actually may be more important than all the noise. In fact, chickens use body language more frequently than oral communication, and it's the basis of good manners in chicken society. If you watch as well as listen, you can translate some of that conversation.

Although you may find this chapter helpful as a spark to your career as a "chicken whisperer," our goal isn't to train you in advanced chicken psychology. We want to emphasize that a basic understanding of natural behaviors of chickens is really important for keeping them healthy. Many chicken illnesses are traced to social discord in the flock or to flock keepers who unknowingly provide a boring environment that stifles natural chicken behaviors. Feather pecking, for example, is a very common behavior problem that can lead to very serious health problems for individual flock members.

Chickens are creatures of habit, and they spend most of their waking hours in devotion to their routines. In this chapter, we give you a rundown of a day in the life of the average hen as she goes through her routine. Next, we discuss what passes for manners in chicken society and present an introduction to Chicken Language 101. The art of fowl courtship wraps up the chapter.

A Day in the Life of a Chicken: The Daily Routine

Chickens tell time and set their routine by the daily cycle of light and darkness. They sense light not only through light-detecting cells in the eyes, but also through special cells in the pineal gland of the brain, which causes hormones to be released through the chicken's body, driving them to do what they do in their daily routines. These sections take a closer look at the typical day and night schedule of a chicken, so you can see when chickens do what they do.

Starting the day and going to work

Most of the flock is awake and at it within an hour of daybreak. Besides breakfast, which is the longest and most important meal of the day, morning is the time for the flock to groom and do stretching exercises. A hen usually performs her beauty rituals, preening and ruffling her feathers, before she takes the first meal of the day. In the morning, chickens spend more time flapping, doing wing stretches, and flying (a little) than at any other time of the day.

Nesting and laying eggs

Chickens normally visit nest boxes sometime between daybreak and 3 p.m. For several hours before a hen lays her egg of the day, her hormones are surging and telling her to prepare. Her pre-laying behavior starts about an hour or two before laying the egg, and during that time, she restlessly investigates several nesting sites before choosing one. She then goes through the motions of building a nest before finally laying the egg. Some hens are harder to please than others, and they reject several perfectly good nests, in our opinion, before settling on just the right one. Older hens aren't as fussy as younger hens, spending less time searching for the best place to lay an egg.

Most hens choose to lay eggs in an enclosed, quiet, dimly lit space that has soft bedding. Cozy is a good word to describe the nest boxes that you've provided.

Even if you've given them convenient and comfy nest boxes, some hens still insist on laying their eggs on the floor every day. Floor-laying is much more common in young hens in the first 4 to 6 weeks of the onset of lay, and the number of floor eggs decreases as a young laying flock gains experience. We don't know all the causes of floor-laying, but we have some control over a few of the known causes. If there is traffic jam — a long line of hens waiting for too few nest boxes — a hen has no choice but to lay her egg on the floor. Also, sometimes a bossy or unfamiliar hen can intimidate another hen and keep her from getting into a box, causing her to lay eggs on the floor.

Hens choose to lay their eggs near other eggs and other birds, which is why they all use one box, even though you've given them several equally comfortable and easily accessible nest boxes. As soon as you see floor eggs, immediately collect them so other birds aren't attracted to lay their eggs on the ground. Leaving eggs lying around on the ground also encourages chickens to pick up the nasty habit of eating eggs.

A hen who is blocked from using her nesting site experiences stress, and, as a consequence, she may lay an abnormal egg. The frustrated hen paces restlessly and calls her distress over and over again. She may hold on to the unlaid egg, keeping it in her shell gland longer than usual. As a result, the retained egg will receive an extra coating of calcium, resulting in an irregular, rough surface on the egg when the hen finally lays it.

To avoid stressing your hens and receiving ugly eggs, provide at least one nest box for every four hens. Place nest boxes in a quieter, lower traffic area of the coop and keep the box stocked with fresh bedding, such as straw or shavings. Refer to *Building Chicken Coops For Dummies* by Todd Brock, David Zook, and Rob Ludlow (John Wiley & Sons, Inc.) for more information about nest boxes.

Preening and dustbathing

The purpose of both preening and dustbathing is to keep feathers in top condition. Consider these activities your chickens' beauty time:

- **Preening:** A bird uses her beak during a preening session to take dabs of oil from the *preen gland,* which is located on her back at the base of the tail. Then, she strokes her feathers to rub in the oil. Well-oiled feathers are more water-resistant, last longer, and are less likely to break. Most backyard chickens keep a twice-a-day preening schedule — morning and evening.

- **Dustbathing:** Most chickens dustbathe once a day, around noon. Every other day, a chicken takes a long dustbath, flopping around in the dirt for 20 minutes or more. The main purpose of dustbathing is to remove stale or excess oil and prevent feathers from becoming matted. Dustbathing discourages, but doesn't eliminate external parasites.

You should provide sand for your backyard chickens to dustbathe in. Sand efficiently removes excess feather oil, and chickens prefer it. See Chapter 13 for a description of a dustbath box that you can build, fill with sand, and delight your chickens. If your chickens have never seen sand before, introduce them to the sand dustbath box gradually by letting them have access to it for a few hours each day for the first week.

Avoiding predators

All day long, birds use their excellent sense of vision to scan the ground and the air for predators. Running away is Plan A for predator avoidance, but if running away fails, and a chicken is caught and held by a predator, playing dead is Plan B. A chicken has no control over the trance-like reflex, which is triggered by any intensely fearful event, including you performing a medical procedure on the chicken. Behaviorists call the reflex *tonic immobility,* and believe that it may be a good strategy, because many predators, especially cats, will stop their attack and walk away as soon as the prey stops moving or doing anything interesting.

If you hold a chicken still on her back for about a minute, for example to do a medical procedure like treat a wound, the event can trigger an episode of tonic immobility where the bird seems asleep or hypnotized. The bird is very afraid of what you're doing. After a minute or two of playing dead, the chicken will get up, and after a few wobbly steps, go about her business as usual. Some people interpret the trance as the bird "knowing that a human is trying to help," but the bird is actually seriously freaked out.

Finding food

Meals are social events for chickens; hens "do lunch" with their friends. Given a choice of locations, chickens choose to eat close together, all at the same time.

Free-range chickens probably spend more than half of their time happily foraging for food, pecking and scratching the ground to expose seeds and dislodge insects and worms from hiding places. Chickens have such a strong urge to forage that birds kept on solid floors or in wire cages with no litter still scratch and peck the floor, even though nothing is there to scratch or peck.

The easy life may not be a sweet life for confined chickens, even pampered pets. Birds fed pellets from a feeder can eat quickly and don't have to spend much time looking for food. By mid-afternoon, most hens have laid their eggs, eaten, and bathed. Now what? Bored birds who have nothing interesting to peck or scratch at often redirect the urge to forage into pecking each other. Feather pecking and the more extreme version of feather pecking, *cannibalism,* happen more frequently in the afternoon than any other time of the day. For more information about the extremely common problems of feather pecking and cannibalism, see Chapter 11.

Flocks that are provided some sort of litter, such as straw, shavings, or sand, have fewer problems with feather pecking. Tossing some scratch feed or veggie scraps to the flock is a great way to keep the birds occupied during the afternoon blahs.

Settling down for the night

Wild fowl relatives of chickens roost on branches in trees to sleep at night, and so do domesticated chickens when they get the opportunity. They seek out good roosting places well before dark, when the afternoon light starts to fade. Roosting seems logical, because birds that sleep high off the ground may run a lower risk of being attacked by predators.

Although your chickens may prefer to act like wild things and roost on tree branches at night, you should provide perches inside their predator-proof coop at night to keep them safe and comfortable. Chickens don't have assigned seats on the perch, and every night a coop drama unfolds as the residents jockey for the best roosting spots. Just before dark, chickens jump up to their chosen perches. They do this altogether, all at once, so that 90 percent of flock members are roosting within a ten-minute period of time. Then, hens jockey for position, with each hen trying to move to a spot in the center, to avoid the exposed and potentially dangerous ends of the perching line. Often, they push their way in between flock mates, knocking at least one of them to a lower perch or to the ground. This shuffling lasts about ten minutes before the hens settle down, packed tightly together on the perch.

If a group of hens has the choice of upper or lower levels of perches, they all choose the higher level, provided that there is room for everybody. A lack of space to accommodate every bird results in *lower-status hens* (the ones near the bottom of the social structure, known as the pecking order) being forced to roost on lower perches or on the ground. Check out the later section, "Pecking order" for more information.

When setting up roosts in your coop, make sure you provide enough perch space — at least 10 inches per bird — for the whole flock to roost on a single perch. Don't expect birds to sleep on different levels of multilevel perches. They only use the lower perches as a ladder to the upper level, because every bird in the flock wants to spend the night on the highest perch. Place nest boxes lower than the perches in a coop, so birds don't sleep in the boxes and mess them up.

Space your coop's perches no more than a foot or two apart, because hens have trouble jumping more than three feet. Hens find going up is easier than coming down, so provide an easy landing. They dislike perfectly round and slender perches.

Chickens are strongly motivated to roost at night, and that feeling stays with them their entire life, even if they never see a perch. In experiments, hens push through heavy doors and brave the wrath of aggressive flock mates to get to a perch, rather than sleep on the ground. Hens housed without perches spend less time resting at night, and they may be more fearful, frustrated, and prone to feather pecking than hens that are able to roost.

Getting Along in the Flock

Chickens were domesticated in and around Thailand several thousand years ago from a wild ancestor, the red junglefowl. What researchers know about the society of chickens was discovered by observing both the red junglefowl, which still exists in the wild, and by observing their domesticated descendants.

Left to their own devices, chickens and red junglefowl naturally form social groups of 4 to 30 birds. A solitary fowl is a sad and lonely creature not likely to live long in a predator-filled world. Most free-range flocks have both male and female members, although sometimes a few bachelor males will form a small band of their own.

Chickens are social creatures and need to be part of a flock. An only-child chicken isn't a happy pet. Four birds make a quorum — the minimum acceptable flock size. Chickens can't live without each other, but flock life isn't always harmonious. These sections describe how a strict social order is maintained in a flock, and point out that chicks learn how to get along in the flock at early age.

Keeping the peace: The rooster's job

A flock is led by a rooster in charge, who defends his harem and his territory from competitors. He is ruler for life, unless a younger, stronger challenger overthrows him. The dominant rooster usually tolerates young males *(cockerels),* until they reach an age and size to be a threat, when he'll try to drive the potential upstarts out of the flock.

Before you start hatching your own chicks, which will be roughly 50 percent male and 50 percent female, think about what you'll do with all those young males, who will grow up to fight each other and wear out the hens. Rehoming roosters is a challenge, because not many people are willing or able to keep them. Eating them or selling them to someone who will eat them are other options to consider.

A ratio of one rooster per 10 to 25 hens is enough to provide the benefits of having a "man around the house." (Trust us, you don't want any more than one rooster for every ten hens, and neither will your hens or your neighbors.) A rooster's main duties include the following:

✔ Fertilize the eggs

✔ Supervise and calm the flock

✔ Guard the flock against predators

✔ Break up fights between hens (hen-on-hen aggression is less frequent when males are present)

Hens seem more at ease when males are around and on the lookout for danger. They lay eggs, whether a rooster is around or not. The rooster's presence does seem to have an effect on the hens' egg production. Pullets raised in mixed-sex flocks mature sooner and begin to lay eggs a couple of weeks earlier than pullets in flocks lacking any roosters. The rooster doesn't need to have physical contact with the hens to have this effect; the girls just need to see him and hear him.

Pecking order

Roosters and hens form separate pecking orders. A *pecking order* is a hierarchy, or power structure, that forms in every chicken flock, in which each bird knows his or her place in the rank. Pecking order is worked out through one-on-one conflict that ranges from dirty looks, to pecks, to all-out battles with beaks and claws. As soon as the pecking order is settled, and every member of the flock knows his or her position in it, fighting is unusual. Hens almost never challenge the authority of males, and aggression between males and females is rare in chicken society.

Relationships are worked out in pairs; strangers fight in twos until each bird has fought all the others. After the first fight, the winner maintains her dominance over the losing bird with pecks or threats, instead of fighting. The combatants remember who won, and generally don't need rematches. A lower-ranking chicken keeps her head down around higher-ranking birds, because raising her head shows disrespect and invites an attack.

Combs (the fleshy crests on the top of chickens' heads) are status symbols — generally, the bigger the comb, the higher the rank. In mixed-breed flocks, hens with straight combs often dominate over birds with other comb types, such as pea combs. Of course, big combs aren't everything, and breed and individual temperament factor into the contest for dominance, too.

Some bird has to be at the bottom of the pecking order. Other birds may continuously peck and harass this poor bird, especially when she is trying to eat. Eventually, as a result of the constant stress and lack of access to food, a low-status bird may stop laying eggs and molt.

Although you can't interfere with the pecking order, you can make things easier for a low-status bird. Make sure the flock has plenty of food and feeder space, and provide a refuge, such as a get-away box or a cave made of straw bales, so a low-status bird can escape the harassment.

Chickens make friends. You may have noticed a special bond between certain pairs of hens, which has nothing to do with their rank in the pecking order. The pairs choose to spend a lot of time together, eating, foraging, and dustbathing side by side. Chickens' memories are short, and they probably will forget their best friends after a two- or three-week separation. If former friends are reunited after a separation of more than a couple of weeks, they'll fight to re-establish the pecking order as if they'd never known each other.

To avoid conflict and stress-related drops in egg production, avoid mixing groups of chickens, especially after pullets have begun to lay eggs. Try not to separate flock members for longer than two weeks.

Sibling rivalry

Chicks have a "terrible twos" phase and make their first aggressive pecks toward their siblings at about 2 weeks of age. It takes another two weeks for them to back down and make submissive gestures to each other. Chicken boys and girls form separate pecking orders between 6 and 10 weeks of age, and during that time they play-fight, but real contact is unusual. The boy chicks are typically more socially advanced than girl chicks of the same age, setting up their social ranks about a week sooner.

You may want to mix chicks from separate hatches in one brooder, for convenience or to manage brooder space. Sooner is better to avoid fighting and injuries. Mixing hatches goes more smoothly if all the chicks are under 2 weeks of age.

Comprehending Chicken Communication

Chickens don't have as large a vocabulary as most other types of birds, but the number and variety of calls is still impressive. Calls can announce important events, such as spotting a predator, laying and nesting, mating, finding food, and issuing threats. Emotions conveyed in calls range from contentment to frustration to fear. These sections point out some common chicken calls and what they mean.

Crowing he's the boss: A rooster

A rooster advertises ownership of his territory with his crow. Other birds can recognize him a long way off by his voice, which is unique to him. He can engage in long-distance crowing duels with males in neighboring territories, and the duelers may size each other up and work differences out with calls rather than physical fights. Everyone knows that roosters crow in the morning, but people who have never kept a rooster may not realize that a good rooster is on duty 24/7, and he *will crow* whenever he is on duty.

 Many people, including our neighbors, want to silence all roosters, especially the ones who duel at 3 a.m. Forget about it. No method — surgical, medical, behavioral, or magical — can reliably stop him from crowing, unless he doesn't survive the procedure.

The flamboyance of the crow overshadows all the other things a rooster has to say.

- **Kuk, kuk, kuk:** When excited, he makes this food call to hens. The more exciting the food, the more excited the call.
- **Gog-gog-gog:** When courting, he makes this rapid stuttering sound, often followed by a low moan. The girls can't resist it.
- **Purr:** This sound calls a hen to a potential nest site.

Clucking away: A hen's chatter

Hens have a lot to talk about and they make a wide variety of noises to express themselves quite clearly. Here is a sampler of hen speech:

- **Qwaaa-qwa-qwa-qwa:** Before laying an egg, the hen repeats this pre-laying call, which sounds similarly to this or a variation on that theme. It's a sound of anticipation, and it can be translated as "Hurry up in that nest box!" or "When's the food going to get here?", depending on the context.
- **Cackle:** This classic sound announces an egg's arrival.
- **Low moan:** When a very hungry hen is shown but not given food, she utters a low moan. Whines and moans signal mild discomforts, like being out in the rain or a minor peck from a pal.
- **Hiss or growl:** A broody hen sitting on eggs or cuddling her chicks may make a hiss or a protest growl if she's disturbed.
- **Purr:** Purring is purring; it means contentment for chickens as well as felines. A hen purrs to reassure her chicks.

Talking among themselves: The sibling chickens

Even before they're hatched, sibling chicks communicate with each other. Believe it or not, developing chick embryos talk to each other from within their eggs, using clicking sounds to encourage the slower growing sibs to catch up or to scold faster growing sibs to slow down a little. All this in-egg chatter helps synchronize the hatch, so that the chicks emerge together at about the same time. The chatter also helps the siblings to bond and recognize each other after they're hatched.

Chicks can recognize mom by the sound of her voice. A mother hen, though, can't tell her chicks apart from other chicks of the same color. Small chicks make several different and easily recognizable calls, including distress cries, pleasure notes, and fear trills.

Understanding basic chicken predator vocabulary

Predators are a life-or-death matter for chickens, so chickens obviously have several calls to describe different types of predators, their proximity, and the level of danger. Here are a few of those calls, normally made by the rooster-in-charge:

- **Kut-kut-kut-kut-RAAH:** This call means a four-legged predator has been spotted.

- **Roar:** A rooster who spies an airborne chicken-killer lets out a roar, and the flock instantly runs and hides. The rooster stands his ground with his head held high. As the menace flies off, he utters a low growl. You can almost see him shaking his fist at the bird.

- **Whine:** If he recognizes that a flying object, maybe a small bird or a plane, isn't dangerous, the rooster will only give it a sideways look and let out a sound just like a puppy's whine.

Many backyard flocks are rooster-less, in which case, the hens look out for each other and make the predator warning and alarm calls. The calls are basically the same as the rooster's, but lack his flair.

Romancing the Hen: Courtship

Late afternoon is chicken romance time. A rooster courts a hen by calling to her and offering food gifts; this behavior is called *tidbitting*. When he has the hen's attention, he *waltzes* — dancing in an arc around her while fluttering one dropped wing. The hen has three choices after viewing this romantic display:

- ✔ **She can avoid him by stepping aside.** If he's a gentleman, he'll take the hint.

- ✔ **She can escape by running away.** He may chase her.

- ✔ **She can crouch, indicating her receptiveness to his advances.** A hen is more likely to crouch for the rooster-in-charge or a rooster she likes. Hens who live without a rooster often crouch for familiar people. Consider it a sign of respect.

What physical qualities do hens want in the ideal mate? Behaviorists studying domesticated chickens and their wild relatives used chicken dating game experiments to answer that question. They discovered that a sexy rooster, in a hen's eyes, has a large, bright red comb, wattles that are perfectly symmetrical and not too large, red eyes, and big spurs. A gorgeous comb is the most important feature, and plumage color matters least to her.

If a hen shows she's interested and crouches, the rooster grasps her at the back of her head with his beak, and mounts, placing both feet on her back. As if on a treadmill, he shuffles his feet on her back, a motion known as *treading*. At the completion of mating, the rooster bends his tail around the hen's tail, places his *cloaca* (the opening in the bottom of the chicken where the digestive tract, reproductive tract, and urinary tract end) next to hers, and deposits the sperm directly into the hen's cloaca.

Even then, the hen can still change her mind. She can decide to keep or eject the sperm. She's more likely to dump the sperm if the rooster is a low-ranking male, and she has the opportunity to upgrade to a higher-ranking rooster.

Some roosters skip the courtship display and don't give the hens a chance to express their receptiveness for mating. These roosters can be extremely aggressive and injure hens with forceful pecks on the head or by tearing the skin on their backs with claws and spurs. Aggressive mating behavior may be hereditary, so we recommend removing a rooster who damages his hens to protect them and future generations. Replace that guy with a rooster who can take the time to court the hens with waltzes and tidbits.

Chapter 4

More Than an Ounce of Prevention: Biosecurity for the Backyard Flock

. . . .

. . . .

*B*iosecurity is a set of practices — things you do every day — that help keep infectious organisms, such as viruses and bacteria, out of your flock. If a disease-causing organism manages to find its way into your flock, the same biosecurity practices can help prevent the spread of the disease between your chickens, or the spread outside your flock to someone else's chickens.

Biosecurity is the most important thing you can do to protect your chickens' health. Why? Infectious diseases of chickens can be extremely difficult to eradicate from a flock after they appear, even if medications or vaccinations are available to control the disease. For many chicken diseases, safe and approved medications or vaccinations aren't available to backyard chicken owners, or if they are available (and affordable), they can't completely remove the disease-causing organism from a flock. The process of ridding a farm from an infectious disease can be expensive, time-consuming, and possibly heart-breaking if the ultimate solution of depopulation is necessary.

In this chapter, we help you recognize the risks of introducing infectious organisms to your flock and help you develop everyday habits to reduce those risks. We also include a section about protecting your birds if you take them to shows or other places where birds gather.

How's Your Biosecurity? Evaluating Your Current Efforts

To see how well you protect your flock already, take the self-assessment in Table 4-1. Read the three items in each row, and circle the item that most closely matches how you manage your flock. (If you don't have a flock yet, choose the item that you can imagine yourself doing, thinking practically.) Then, add up the number of items you chose in each column.

Table 4-1	Rate Your Biosecurity	
Column A	*Column B*	*Column C*
I have written down my biosecurity plan, and I show the plan to anyone who helps me care for my birds and discuss it with them.	I've thought about biosecurity, and I stick to some common-sense rules that I made for myself and anyone else who helps me take care of my birds.	What's biosecurity?
My chickens are all about the same age.	I have different ages of chickens, but I keep chicks in separate pens from adults at least 30 feet apart.	My chickens of all ages (chicks and adults) have contact with each other.
I use an "all in-all out" system. I got all my chickens at the same time. I won't get more chickens until the ones I have now are gone.	If I get new chickens, I keep them separate from my other birds for 30 days before mixing them together.	When I get new chickens, I introduce them right away to my flock.
My chickens are kept inside a building where they rarely or never have contact with other animals, including wild birds.	My chickens are kept inside a fence or pen outdoors, and they may have contact with wild birds.	My birds are free to roam, which includes the neighbors' yards.
I get all my chickens as hatching eggs or day-old chicks from flocks that participate in the National Poultry Improvement Plan or another health certification program.	I get my chickens as hatching eggs or chicks from different places. I don't always know the health status of the flock they came from.	I look for a good deal. The chickens I bring home can be adults, chicks, or hatching eggs, from all kinds of places, perhaps even swap meets and auctions.

Column A	*Column B*	*Column C*
I clean and disinfect empty pens, waterers, and feeders and let them stay empty and unused for at least three days before using them for other chickens.	I clean empty pens, waterers, and feeders, and then use them for chickens right away.	My pens are never empty, and I never get a chance to clean and disinfect pens, waterers, or feeders.
My chickens stay home. They never leave my place.	I take chickens to shows, auctions, sales, or swap meets, but I sell them there, and they don't come home with me again.	I take chickens to shows, auctions, sales, or swap meets, and they come back home with me.
I clean and disinfect transport coops after using them to bring chickens to or take chickens away from my place.	I don't disinfect my transport coops, but I don't share them with anyone else or put anyone else's birds in them.	I don't clean transport coops, and I don't mind sharing them with anyone who needs them.
I don't allow visitors to see my birds, unless they have a really good reason. I don't allow anyone who has been in contact with other birds in the last three days to have contact with my birds.	I rarely have visitors, and when people do visit, I ask them to clean their hands and shoes before they visit my birds.	I have many visitors, including poultry owners. I may even host a farm tour or a swap meet at my place. Visitors aren't asked to clean their hands or shoes.
I only have chickens, and no other types of birds at my place.	I keep other types of birds besides chickens, but each type of bird is kept separate.	I have all types of birds, maybe even pet birds, like parrots and finches, or other poultry, such as ducks, and they may be kept in the same pen or room.
Column A Score: ___	Column B Score: ___	Column C Score: ___

After you add your scores, look at each column's final score. The items in Column A represent best practices for backyard chicken keeping, but they may not be practical for many backyard flock keepers. Column B contains compromises or middle-of-the-road practices that most backyard flock owners can practically do. The last column, Column C, describes keeping chickens with little thought to biosecurity.

If your Column A score is higher than the scores for the other columns, you're doing a really good job of limiting your flock's risk of encountering disease-causing organisms. Most likely, however, you circled more items in Column B than in Column A or C, and you've thought about protecting your flock, but you may not have considered biosecurity as seriously as you can. Think about whether any of the practices in Column A are practical for you to adopt. Finally, if you scored heavy on the Column C items, your flock is at high risk for encountering disease-causing organisms, if it isn't affected by them already. Biosecurity can be simple and practical; read on, and see if you can adopt some of the common-sense precautions we discuss later in this chapter.

Recognizing How Disease Is Spread in Chicken Flocks

Disease can spread to your chickens in many ways, but bringing other birds into the flock is enemy number one for backyard flock biosecurity; in fact, it's the most common way for infectious organisms to invade your flock. People who are constantly moving and handling things are also pretty good at tracking germs around on their bodies (particularly their hands), and also on clothes and shoes. Infectious organisms frequently lurk on stuff that a chicken (especially a sick chicken) has had the opportunity to mess up, like coops and cars. Flock keepers know that chickens quickly take advantage of opportunities to explore and mess up objects in their environments!

Basically an infectious disease can be spread from flock to flock by the following methods. This list is organized in "worry order" — roughly, not exactly. The big risks that you should worry about and focus on avoiding are toward the top of the list.

- ✔ A live bird or fertile egg infected with the disease-causing organism. Infected chickens may appear sick, or they may appear healthy but carry the organism without showing any signs of it.
- ✔ Dead bird carcasses.
- ✔ People carrying the organism on their bodies, shoes, or clothing.
- ✔ Non-living stuff contaminated with the organism, such as coops, egg cartons, or vehicles.

✔ Other animals, including insects, carrying the organism in or
on their bodies.

✔ Contaminated feed or feed bags.

✔ Contaminated water, such as surface drainage water.

✔ Airborne organisms.

The following sections take a closer look at the three top worries:
birds, people, and stuff that birds (or bird poop) has touched. The
other things on the preceding list may be the source of an infectious organism, but those ways of spreading them aren't as easy
or common.

The big risk: The new chicken (or the new egg)

Bringing new chickens home is the biggest risk a flock owner can
take. Chickens are factories for producing infectious organisms
that infect other chickens. Usually, viruses and bacteria that like to
live in chickens and make them sick multiply rapidly and grow well
only in chickens, and not in other types of animals. For example,
a chicken infected with Marek's disease virus may produce and
shed from its skin a *billion* virus particles a day! On the other hand,
when quail become infected with Marek's disease virus, which is
rare, they produce few virus particles compared to infected chickens. The virus doesn't multiply in people at all.

Think about bringing the example chicken with its billion Marek's
disease virus particles to your place. Then think about a fellow
flock owner visiting your place on the same day, carrying a few
Marek's disease virus particles in the dust in her hair. Which of
those two, the infected chicken or the dusty-haired visitor, is more
likely to be the source of Marek's disease introduced to your flock
that day? (If you are interested in reading more about Marek's disease, check out Chapter 12.)

The ways that infections are transmitted between chickens are
different, depending on the type of infection. Viruses that cause
chicken respiratory diseases usually multiply in the respiratory
system: the air passages, lungs, or air sacs. The infected chicken
coughs or sneezes, spewing the virus particles into the air or spat-
tering nearby surfaces and flock mates with virus-laden mucous.
Infectious organisms that cause diarrhea usually multiply inside
the cells lining the intestines and spread in the poop. Organisms
that invade the hen's reproductive tract may also invade her eggs,
infecting her chicks even before they're hatched.

A sick chicken is an obvious source of illness for a flock. Two sneakier ways that infectious organisms can enter a flock are hatching eggs and carrier chickens.

Fertile hatching eggs as a source of disease

Bringing home, incubating, and hatching fertile eggs is a fun and inexpensive way to obtain new birds from far-away flocks. However, fertile eggs can be a source of infection for a flock, if the hens that laid the eggs passed an infection through the eggs to their chicks. Avian encephalomyelitis, mycoplasmosis, and pullorum disease are some examples of egg-transmitted diseases of chickens, which we talk about in more detail in Chapter 12.

The carrier chicken (not at all like a carrier pigeon!)

A troublesome concept in poultry health is the *carrier state*. Many types of organisms that cause diseases in chickens can live hidden within a chicken, causing no signs of illness, or causing signs that are so mild they aren't noticed by anyone. Maybe, sometime in the past, the carrier chicken was sick and recovered from the disease, but the organism moved in permanently. The carrier chicken appears healthy but harbors the organism for a long time, often the rest of her life, and it may spread the infection to flock mates without anyone being aware of it.

To name just a few, the following are some chicken diseases that can result in a carrier state:

✔ Fowl cholera

✔ Infectious coryza

✔ Infectious laryngotracheitis

✔ Marek's disease

✔ Mycoplasmosis

Chapter 12 discusses these diseases in more detail.

The effect of stress on a carrier chicken can be disastrous. Stress has a negative effect on the immune system of any animal. Chicken stress comes in many forms, including hot weather, cold weather, bad food, bullying flock mates, and moving to a new home. Put a carrier chicken in one of those less-than-comfortable situations, and while the chicken's immune system is not at its best, the previously hidden organism may rear its ugly head — the chicken becomes sick. In stressful times, the carrier chicken is especially infectious, because it often produces large numbers of organisms to share with its flock mates and has the means (sneezing or diarrhea, for example) to spread it.

The other risks: People, other animals, and equipment

Your flock can be at risk from other sources as well. People can haul infectious organisms from place to place unaware that their bodies, clothes, and shoes are contaminated with them. Other animals (dogs, cats, and rats, to name some common culprits) can carry the organisms on their skin and fur. Objects that have been used to hold, feed, water, or clean up after infected chickens are also likely to be covered with infectious organisms.

What's the chance that these contaminated people, animals, or equipment will be the source of infection for a flock? It depends mostly on the ability of the organism to survive off the chicken during its journey from one chicken to the next. Some organisms are very durable and can survive in the environment for months to years. Others, especially some respiratory disease viruses, are relatively wimpy and only last outside the chicken for a few hours or a few days. Some conditions are more favorable than others; generally, moist, cool, dark, and dirty environments help disease organisms last longer. Table 4-2 contains some chicken diseases and the typical environmental survival times of the organisms that cause them.

Table 4-2	How Long Organisms Survive in the Environment
Disease	*Survival time*
Avian tuberculosis	Years
Marek's disease	Months to years
Coccidiosis	Months
Infectious bursal disease	Months
Newcastle disease	Days to weeks
Infectious coryza	Hours to days
Mycoplasmosis	Hours to days

Chicken disease-causing germs can stay alive on clothing, on equipment, and in the environment for hours to years, depending on the how tough the organism is. That's why it's really important to clean hands, clothes, shoes, and equipment after working with chickens, to prevent spreading disease. We give cleaning and disinfection tips in Chapter 5. Keeping other animals (pets and pests) out of the chicken pen is also an important disease control measure.

Potential critters in chicken feed

Chickens may be exposed to disease-causing organisms in their food. Common feed ingredients that come from animals, such as meat, bones, or blood, are good sources of nutritious protein or minerals, but they're likely to contain infectious organisms, such as *Salmonella* bacteria, unless the ingredients are well-cooked.

Furthermore, rodents and insects are very determined in their efforts to get an easy, nutritious meal of chicken feed, by chewing and squeezing their way into feed sacks, storage bins, and chicken houses. Rodent diners are generous tippers, leaving behind droppings that may contain disease-causing organisms they harbor, particularly *Salmonella* bacteria. Rodent and insect control is a constant challenge for flock owners, but fighting the battle is important for the health of the flock. We get into more detail about keeping feed fresh and pest-free in Chapter 5.

To reduce the risk of bacterial contamination of chicken feed, many feed manufacturers produce vegetarian diets for chickens, avoiding any ingredients made from animals. Also, the process that manufacturers use to make pelleted or crumbled feed involves cooking, which kills the bacteria that may have been in the raw ingredients. Home-made, whole-grain, or table-scrap diets for chickens may not be as well-cooked.

Extreme biosecurity: A visit to a commercial poultry farm

Few people have seen the inside of a modern commercial poultry farm where a high level of biosecurity is practiced, and that's by design. Commercial poultry producers want to prevent people from introducing infectious diseases that may harm the flock or the flock's ability to produce eggs or meat efficiently. Generally only the birds' caretakers, the few people who maintain and fix the building and equipment, and an occasional outside consultant, such as the flock veterinarian, are allowed to visit the farm.

Because you may not have the opportunity to see it for yourself, we describe what you may see if you were invited to visit a high-biosecurity poultry farm, specifically, a layer farm producing eggs. First, when you set your appointment, you'll be asked to stay away from other birds (including pet birds such as parrots) for at least 72 hours prior to your visit. As you approach the farm on the day of your appointment, you see a fence that completely surrounds the farm, preventing people, dogs, and other animals from approaching the poultry houses. The spaces between the poultry houses are tidy, just gravel and short mowed grass, and nothing else, to discourage rodents and insects from hiding nearby. All the windows and the ventilation openings of the houses are covered in screens to prevent wild birds and insects from entering.

At the farm gate is a reception office, where you meet the farm manager. She asks you to sign a visitor log, and then she describes the *shower in-shower out* procedure and shows you the door to the changing room. You undress and walk into a shower room, soap and rinse your entire body, and exit through a different door in the shower room. On the other side, a clean pair of overalls and rubber boots, and a disposable hair net, surgical mask, and latex gloves await you. You put on all these items and walk out the door to the path that takes you to the poultry houses. You realize that you're quite uncomfortable wearing all that gear.

The manager escorts you on your tour, describing the farm as you walk. She tells you that you won't be allowed to enter the houses with the chickens, but you can view them through the windows in the doors to the houses. At the door to each house is a boot wash station, which is used each time a caretaker enters and leaves the house. Each of several houses on the farm holds about 100,000 laying hens. Most of the chores (feeding, watering, egg collecting, and waste removal) are done automatically by machines, not only to make the work easier, but also to reduce the number of people who must have contact with the chickens and possibly spread disease to them.

The manager goes on to describe the all-in, all-out system on this farm. An empty house is filled with young ready-to-lay hens all at once, and the hens stay there until their best laying days are done, when all of the chickens leave the house at the same time. After the birds leave the house, it's thoroughly cleaned, disinfected, and left empty for two weeks before new birds are brought in. The new, young hens arrive in cleaned and disinfected transport coops.

The farm has a truck wash station, where each vehicle that arrives, usually a truck delivering feed or taking away eggs, must be washed when it enters, and washed again when it leaves the farm. Before being loaded into feed trucks, the feed was sampled and tested to make sure it wasn't contaminated with disease-causing bacteria or mold toxins.

At the end of your visit, you exit through the changing room, leaving behind the coveralls and boots for cleaning and disinfection, and the disposable hair net, mask, and gloves for incineration. You shower again, change into your own clothes, and rejoin the farm manager in the office. Before leaving the farm, you ask a few more questions, including whether all commercial layer farms are managed the same way as this one. She tells you that all producers don't follow the same disease control practices, but most do some of the measures you've seen here. You say good-bye to the manager, thanking her for an eye-opening visit.

To avoid food-transmitted chicken illnesses, use only commercial pelleted or crumbled feed. Chapter 6 has more information about chicken feed choices. If you feed table scraps to your chickens, make sure foods that contain meat, eggs, or dairy products are well cooked before feeding them.

Designing Your Biosecurity Plan

The parts of your biosecurity plan, whether you write the plan down or keep the rules in your head, should include things you do to keep out disease, and the ways you do your daily chores to prevent disease from spreading between your birds. No matter whether your chickens stay home or go to shows, your biosecurity plan should address what to do. This section can help you get started.

Keeping out disease

As we mention earlier in this chapter, new birds are the biggest risk for introducing an infectious disease to your flock. We recommend that you do a little homework so that you can have the best chance of bringing home healthy birds to start your flock or to keep it going. These steps can help improve your chance of bringing home healthy birds:

1. **Be choosy about the sources of your new birds.**

2. **Know how to recognize signs of illness and examine a bird in order to select the healthiest individuals.**

3. **Isolate the new birds so that you can detect problems before you move them permanently into their new home or let them join your existing flock.**

These sections walk you through these steps in greater depth to make the selection process easier and increase the likelihood that you pick healthy birds.

Assessing the risk of sources of birds

Choosing the safest sources of healthy new birds for your flock can be confusing. Notice we say "safest" and not "completely safe." We can't promise you fool-proof selection, but we can offer three tips to help you choose birds from places least likely to share an infectious disease with your flock: youngest birds, closed flock, and known health status.

✔ **Youngest birds:** Older birds have had more time and opportunity to encounter an infectious disease in their flock or their home environment. Hatching eggs and day-old chicks are safer to bring home than growing and adult birds. This tip doesn't prevent you from bringing home egg-transmitted diseases, however.

✔ **Closed flock:** People who keep *closed* flocks don't bring new birds into their flocks and their birds never leave home and return. Having a closed flock limits the chance of introducing an infectious disease. Year after year, closed flock owners raise chicks from parent birds that live at the same site.

To know whether a potential source flock is closed, you need to ask the flock owner. Owners of closed flocks usually appreciate you asking about it, and are happy to tell you how long they've managed their flock that way. The riskiest sources are bird dealers, auctions, and flea markets, where birds are constantly moving in, mixing, and moving out. That's asking for trouble.

✔ **Known health status:** While you're talking to the flock owner, find out about the flocks' health status. Is the flock enrolled in a health certification program, such as the National Poultry Improvement Plan? What diseases does the flock owner test for on a regular basis? Is the flock owner aware of any infectious disease problem in the flock? Of course, you or the flock owner can't be certain about the absence of every infectious chicken disease, but the more you know about the flock's health status, the better.

Choosing healthy birds

If you bring home fertile eggs for hatching, choose and incubate eggs that are clean and intact, without cracks or chips in the shells. Washing or dipping eggs in a sanitizing solution can remove disease-causing organisms from the outside of the shell without harming hatchability, but it doesn't remove infectious organisms from the eggs' contents.

When choosing chicks, take a look first at how well the chicks have been kept at the store. Is the bedding relatively clean and dry? Do the chicks have an adequate heat source, or are they huddled for warmth? Then, pick the larger, more robust chicks that seem to be alert, eating, drinking, and moving around well. They should have clear eyes and nostrils, and fluffy down. Beaks, legs, and toes should not look crooked or twisted. A chick's navel should be dry and not protrude from the abdomen.

Bringing home growing or adult birds is the riskiest option, from the perspective of keeping disease out of your flock. Avoid buying adult birds sight-unseen without a veterinary examination and health certificate. We suggest that you read Chapter 7 and do a thorough examination of an older bird before you decide to bring her home to introduce to your flock. Doing so can help you avoid the obviously sick birds, but keep in mind that you won't be able to *see* the healthy-looking chicken that is carrying an infectious organism. If you have the means and opportunity to test the bird for infectious diseases, the best time to perform the tests is before you bring her home.

Bring home new birds in your own clean and disinfected plastic carriers or transport coops. Cardboard boxes are okay for chicks, as long as they're brand new. Hatching eggs should be transported in new packing material or clean and disinfected plastic egg trays.

Introducing new birds to your flock

When adding new birds to your flock, use the *30-30 isolation rule.* New birds should be isolated for at least 30 days before you mix them with your existing flock, at least 30 feet away from any other birds. Waiting 30 days gives plenty of time for most infectious diseases to appear, if one is incubating in the new group of chickens. The separation distance of 30 feet is somewhat arbitrary, but it's based on the imagined "sneeze zone" of a chicken, plus several feet as a safety factor. You should choose a relatively closed isolation place, such as a shed or a barn, rather than an open-air pen, where you don't intend to keep your home-raised chicks or growing birds later on.

Take care of the isolated birds after you've tended to the rest of your flock. The isolation place should have its own feeders, waterers, and cleaning tools, like pitchforks and wheelbarrows, that you don't use anywhere else on your place, unless you clean and disinfect them first. Dispose of the litter and other waste from the isolation place in a separate location from manure from the rest of the flock. Having running water available nearby is really helpful to wash your hands before and after taking care of the isolated birds. If running water isn't nearby, keep a bottle of hand sanitizer in a handy spot.

Some people set up foot baths filled with disinfectant near the entrance to the isolation area. Doing so seems like a good idea, but foot baths are difficult to maintain and getting people to use them properly is even harder, so we're not fans of foot baths and don't recommend them. We suggest either dedicating a pair of boots to use only in the isolation area, or washing boots with soap and water after doing isolation area chores.

Treat older birds for external and internal parasites (lice, mites, and worms) at the start of the isolation period, and repeat the treatment two weeks later, halfway through. For chicks, external parasite treatment shouldn't be necessary. We provide more information on treatments for external and internal parasites in Chapter 13 and in the appendix. The start of the isolation period is also the time to vaccinate the birds, if you vaccinate your flock, and if the birds are the appropriate age for your vaccination program. See Chapter 16 for information about chicken vaccinations.

When a bird becomes sick during the isolation period, immediately remove it from the rest of group. Doing so may sound harsh, but unless you're certain that the cause of illness isn't transmissible, euthanizing the sick bird is the safest thing to do; don't risk the rest of your flock with a sick newcomer. You can get the most information about the problem by submitting the bird to a veterinary diagnostic laboratory for analysis. If you aren't able to submit the bird to experts for diagnosis, you may perform the postmortem yourself, or at least dispose of the bird in a way that doesn't spread disease. We talk about euthanasia and disposal in Chapter 18, and submitting a bird for diagnosis or performing a do-it-yourself chicken postmortem in Chapter 15.

Testing the birds for infectious diseases near the end of the isolation period, but before you release them from isolation, is an excellent idea, although you may not find it feasible. If all goes well, and the new birds pass the isolation period in fine health, examine them once more and make sure they're looking great before letting them join the rest of the flock

Developing biosecurity habits in your daily chore routine

Biosecurity practices are easier if they become habits — things you do routinely every day without thinking about it much. One habit that costs nothing and is feasible for any flock keeper is doing chores in order of youngest to oldest birds.

Getting rid of a disease after it enters a *multi-age flock* — one where chicks and older birds are kept together — is very frustrating, if not impossible. The adult birds pass their infections to each new batch of chicks, and the cycle continues, generation after generation, and year after year.

To avoid that vicious cycle, most large commercial farms use an *all-in, all-out* system, and keep only one age group on one farm at a time. Chickens are hatched in one place, they grow up in another, and they may be moved yet again for the production stage. An all-in, all-out system is possible for a family raising one batch of *broilers* (meat-type chickens) each year, but it's not practical for backyard flock keepers who want to breed and raise their own birds.

If raising and breeding your own chickens is your goal, what can you do? You can plan your daily chicken care chores in order of your youngest to your oldest birds. Ideally, use a separate set of tools, such as feed scoop, pitchfork, and manure bucket for each age group, but you can clean them before using them with another group. When you finish taking care of one age group, wash your hands and clean your boots before moving on to the next group. Take care of isolated and sick birds last. Before repeating your route for next chore time, put on a clean set of work clothes and boots. Better yet, shower and change clothes. For example, chores on a multi-age backyard flock may proceed like this on a beautiful morning:

1. **Check the incubator and then the hatcher.**

   You have hatchlings!

2. **Move the fluffy new chicks to the brooder and tend to the other baby birds.**

3. **Feed and water the young birds in the grow-out pen.**

   Everyone looks great.

4. **Feed, water, and collect eggs from the laying hens.**

   Good morning, girls!

5. **Check on the new birds in the isolation area.**

   You're happy to see that they've finished their feed and look well. They're a rare breed you've always wanted, but you couldn't find until last week.

6. **Doctor the poor old hen in the hospital pen.**

   You don't know how she got that big cut on her back.

7. **Done with morning chores, wash your boots and hands before getting your coffee.**

   This afternoon, you'll wear a clean set of clothes to do the rounds again.

Considering biosecurity for show chickens

The best way to avoid disease problems at chicken shows is not to attend them. For some chicken owners, though, raising beautiful show birds and then enjoying poultry show competition are the main reasons to keep chickens. If you decide you really want to go, we give you a few suggestions to reduce the risk of picking up an infectious disease at a chicken show. Have fun, but be careful.

Can you take birds to the show, but not return home with them? Doing so is the safest way to go; take only birds that you intend to sell at the show. If you can't, these sections give you a few more ideas to cut your risk.

Before the show

The healthiest-looking birds in the best condition are the ones that win the highest honors at a poultry show. They're in excellent condition because they've been fed well and kept in a clean and comfortable environment. They're also, because of their superior condition, less susceptible to disease than birds that haven't had those advantages. Any bird that isn't the picture of vibrant health should stay home.

Keep the following tips in mind before you attend the show:

- ✔ **Plan ahead and check the show's health rules to understand what tests or health certifications are required.** It may take some time to set up an appointment with your veterinarian or flock inspector to get tests done and receive results or to obtain a health certificate or movement permit. Show rules may prohibit or require certain vaccinations. Consider setting up a vaccination program for your exhibition flock (see Chapter 16).

- ✔ **Avoid unnecessary stress for your birds.** Choose shows that last for no more than a day or two that are held during spring or fall, when the weather isn't likely to be too cold or too hot. Put show birds in exhibition-size cages several days before you go, so they can be accustomed to the smaller space and perhaps strange feeding and watering cups.

- ✔ **Clean and disinfect your transport coops and carriers before you load up your birds to go.** Avoid using cardboard boxes or wooden boxes that you can't properly clean and disinfect.

At the show

Our advice is to be a fussy exhibitor at the show. When you *coop-in* (put your birds in their cages at the show), take a look at the competition. Your birds' neighbors should appear healthy and active. They should not have runny eyes or nostrils or scabs or swellings on their heads, and there should not be several loose droppings in the cage. Don't be afraid to report birds that don't appear healthy to show officials. You may need to be persistent, but polite, to get busy show officials to investigate a sick bird and ask the owner to remove it from the show. Most of your fellow exhibitors will support you and appreciate the effort.

Remember these warnings while at the show:

▶ **Don't touch other exhibitors' birds.** Poultry exhibitors consider it bad sportsmanship for you to handle their birds. We think it's also unsanitary.

▶ **Bring and use your own cage cups for feed and water.** Don't share cage cups, feed scoops, or watering cans with other exhibitors.

Returning home

If you must return home with show birds, isolate them as if they were new birds; we describe how to do this in "Introducing new birds to your flock," earlier in this chapter. You may keep a separate isolation area just for your show birds during the entire show season. Don't put returning birds that show signs of respiratory illness while in isolation back in the flock. Check and/or treat for external parasites (lice and mites) before letting show birds rejoin the flock.

Chapter 5

Keeping the Flock Clean and Comfortable

In This Chapter

▶ Reducing disease-causing organisms with cleaning and disinfecting

▶ Offering your flock a healthy environment

*H*appiness is a clean pen. If the flock's response to a freshly cleaned pen isn't an expression of sheer pleasure, we have completely misread the situation. We're sure you, like us, have heard the hens' excited clucking, seen them playing keep-away with the bright clean straw and exploring all the corners of an old coop as if it's brand new, and watched them sip contentedly from the sparkling clean waterer. They clearly appreciated your efforts.

This chapter isn't about the emotional life of chickens; it's about keeping the flock clean and comfortable. No one likes to clean (okay, we've met a few people who *say* they do), but cleaning is an extremely important part of keeping the flock healthy — and happy. In this chapter, we try to make applying the elbow grease a tad easier.

Have you thought about what you'll do with the flock when the weather turns uncomfortable or downright nasty? We also share some ideas about the bad weather to help you prepare.

Cleaning and Disinfecting (C&D) 101

The aim of cleaning and disinfecting is to kill as many disease-causing organisms as practically possible. In the business, it's known as *C&D*.

The steps of C&D are the same, whether you're working with a small item like a transport coop, or a large area, such as a shed or barn. The four cleaning steps are dry cleaning, washing, rinsing, and drying, followed by the four disinfection steps: application, contact time, rinsing, and downtime.

For routine daily or weekly chores, such as cleaning feeding pans or waterers, the first four steps — dry cleaning, cleaning with soap and water, rinsing, and drying — are usually sufficient. The following situations are when you need to pull out the full eight-step C&D process:

- ✔ Before you restock an empty pen

- ✔ Before you use equipment, such as transport coops, or vehicles that have been used for someone else's birds

- ✔ After a sick chicken leaves the hospital pen or after quarantined birds are released from isolation

- ✔ Before you put young birds in an area where adult birds had been kept previously

- ✔ After chickens have been removed from an area due to an infectious disease outbreak

- ✔ Before and after processing eggs or chicken meat for human consumption

Beginning with construction

Make C&D easy on yourself from the start. When you're planning to build your backyard coop, imagine yourself cleaning it. The coop may be just the right size for your hens, but if you can't reach all corners to clean, you'll later regret the design.

 Choose construction materials that you can easily clean and disinfect. Stick with nonporous materials, such as plastic, sheet metal, and wire, which are easier to clean. Avoid using porous materials, such as wood, fabric, and rope, if you can, because they're next to impossible to disinfect.

Most flock keepers use wood to build coops, because wood is relatively inexpensive, readily available, and easy to work with, but it's difficult to keep clean. If you must use wood, choose a solid wood, rather than particle board, plywood, or composite wood materials, and then paint the wood or use another type of sealant. (Check out *Building Chicken Coops For Dummies* by Todd Brock, David Zook, and Rob Ludlow [John Wiley & Sons, Inc.] for more information about building your coops.)

Grasping the art of cleaning

Cleaning is by far the most important step in the C&D process. If you do it right, cleaning removes more than 90 percent of disease-causing organisms. On the other hand, if you don't do the cleaning step well, the disinfectant won't work, and you'll have wasted time and money. Follow these four steps to make sure you're cleaning in detail:

1. **Dry clean to collect the big stuff.**

   Dry cleaning, in this case, doesn't involve delicate fabrics; it involves effort — scraping, shoveling, sweeping, or vacuuming to remove most of the debris that you easily see. A muck bucket or wheelbarrow can help cart the stuff away for disposal as far away from the chickens as possible.

   Although a hand-held or backpack lawn blower may seem like an easy way to clean up, it's actually a quick, effective germ dispersal tool! Don't use it for chicken-house cleaning. If an area is especially dusty (as chicken coops usually are), use a hose to wet surfaces down with water before starting to sweep.

2. **Wash with soap and water.**

   After dry cleaning, the area or item probably won't be visibly clean, because of stubborn dirt or caked-on droppings. Pre-soaking with warm, soapy water for a couple of hours can soften the gunk and make the washing job easier. Whenever possible, use hot water. A pressure washer with detergent is very effective at removing caked-on droppings and for cleaning porous surfaces, like wood.

   Our favorite backyard flock clean-up tools are a 5-gallon bucket with a handle and a long-handled scrub brush with extra stiff bristles — where you shop, it may be referred to as a *long-handled fender brush.*

3. **Rinse with clean water.**

   After rinsing, surfaces should be visibly clean. If not, go back to Step 2.

4. **Allow surfaces to air dry completely.**

   Take advantage of a free, natural disinfectant, if you have it — ultraviolet (UV) light — and put washed and rinsed objects in the sun to dry. Wait, if you can, until all surfaces are dry before moving on to the disinfection steps, which we discuss next, because your disinfectant will work better.

Getting a hold on disinfection

Think of disinfection as a safety net, to kill organisms that you can't see that escaped your washing process. Disinfection methods can be physical, such as heat and UV light, or chemical. Stick to these steps to disinfect your coops and other important areas:

1. **Apply the disinfectant.**

   Don't just sprinkle it; thoroughly wet the item or area, if you're using a chemical disinfectant. A 1-gallon garden sprayer works well for small flock jobs. Submerge small things in a plastic container filled with disinfectant solution.

2. **Allow adequate contact time.**

   Most disinfectants don't instantaneously kill organisms, so contact time is really important for the disinfectant to make an impact. Read the label to find the required contact time (or *dwell time*) for a chemical disinfectant. You may need to reapply the disinfectant in order to keep the item or area wet for the required contact time.

3. **Thoroughly rinse off chemical disinfectants.**

   Like other animals, chickens can suffer from chemical burns or skin irritation if they have contact with disinfectant solutions. Thoroughly rinse the disinfectant off with clean water before putting the item or area back in service for your flock.

4. **Allow all items to completely dry, and let clean areas rest for a while.**

   Things and places that have been cleaned and disinfected should have a period of downtime afterwards. As we mention in Chapter 4, many disease-causing organisms only last hours or a few days in the environment, so downtime may buy you some time, while any remaining organisms fade away. Downtime is particularly important when you C&D between groups of chickens; if possible, leave a clean coop, barn, or pen empty for at least two weeks before you bring in the new flock.

The perfect disinfectant kills all types of infectious organisms, and it's inexpensive, easy to use, noncorrosive, and completely nontoxic for humans and animals. Unfortunately the perfect disinfectant doesn't exist! They all have advantages and disadvantages; we try to help you choose a good one for your situation in the following sections.

Physical disinfectants

Heat and ultraviolet light are two physical disinfection methods that may be practical for you.

   ✔ **Heat disinfection:** This method is probably most useful to backyard flock keepers as a way to disinfect food for chickens, such as cooking discarded eggs or table scraps, but if you want to steam clean your coop, go for it! Most bacteria and viruses are inactivated by moist heat above 160 degrees

Fahrenheit (70 degrees Celsius). Boiling for 20 minutes ought to do the job on most poultry disease-causing organisms. On the flip side, freezing slows organisms down, but it's not a reliable method of disinfection.

✔ **Ultraviolet light:** You can find UV light in sunlight or generated by specialized lamps. UV light kills disease-causing organisms, but it acts only on surfaces of objects or on particles in the air, and it can't penetrate even a thin film or into cracks and crevices. Six hours of exposure to full sunlight can inactivate many types of bacteria and viruses clinging to smooth surfaces. You can disinfect small quantities of water in about the same time, by setting water-filled transparent bottles in full sunlight.

Chemical disinfectants

Chemical disinfectants kill a wide variety of disease-causing organisms, but some types of organisms are easier to kill than others. Bacteria and some viruses succumb rapidly to most disinfectants, although other viruses and fungal spores are tougher. Some parasites, like *coccidia* (see Chapter 13), laugh at most common disinfectants and go about their business.

Dozens of disinfectants are available for backyard flock keepers to use, although knowing which one is the best choice for the job can be confusing. They vary in their effectiveness against certain types of organisms, ease of use, toxicity, corrosiveness, and cost.

To make your choice easier, we suggest you use household bleach, which is simple to use, very effective at killing germs, and inexpensive. Household bleach (5.25 percent sodium hypochlorite) inactivates a wide range of disease-causing organisms and has low toxicity when diluted and used properly. Table 5-1 gives common dilutions of household bleach and their uses.

Table 5-1   Recommended Household Bleach Solutions

Use	Bleach Amount Per Gallon of Water
Disinfecting drinking water	⅛ teaspoon (eight drops)
Controlling slime in drinkers and waterers	¼ teaspoon (16 drops)
Submerging small items; spraying surfaces; wiping incubators, egg trays, and food-preparation surfaces	1 tablespoon

(continued)

Table 5-1 *(continued)*

Use	Bleach Amount Per Gallon of Water
General disinfection for non-food contact surfaces	¼ cup

*Use regular, unscented household bleach with a concentration of 4 to 6 percent sodium hypochlorite

If you want more information about other types of chemical disinfectants, we list the main categories, examples of each type, and their advantages and disadvantages in the appendix.

Concentrates, which you dilute in water before using, are more economical than ready-to-use disinfectant solutions. Many disinfectants are quickly inactivated by dirt or time, so don't use leftover disinfectant solutions that you've prepared from concentrate. Instead, mix a fresh batch just before you intend to use it. Also mix up a fresh batch if the solution starts to look dirty while you're applying it, because it's probably not working well anymore.

Safely using and disposing of disinfectants

Read the label before you purchase a disinfectant to see if it's right for your job, and read it again before you use it, in order to mix and use it safely. The label also informs you of safe ways to dispose of the product after you've finished the job.

All disinfectants sold in the United States must be registered with the Environmental Protection Agency (EPA). The registration number listed on the product label shows that the EPA has reviewed the product and that it can be used with minimal risk to people, other animals, or the environment, if the label directions are followed properly.

Along with directions for mixing and using the disinfectant, the product label also describes potential hazards to people or animals and actions to take to reduce those hazards, such as wearing gloves or goggles. Specific signal words are used to indicate the degree of hazard. From least harmful to most harmful, the signal words are the following: Caution, Warning, Danger, and Danger-Poison. The label tells you whether the product is potentially hazardous to fish, wildlife, plants, or water sources, and provides ways to use the product and avoid damage to the environment. Storage and disposal instructions for the product and for the empty container are also written on the label.

What do you do if the label has come off, or if it's unreadable? Go online and check the EPA website at `http://iaspub.epa.gov/apex/pesticides/f?p=PPLS:1`, or type the product name and label information into a search engine.

Treat your disinfectants as toxic accidents waiting to happen. Protect the health of people and other animals by keeping the following points in mind:

- ✔ Store disinfectants in their original containers in a cool, dark place, away from pets and children.

- ✔ Don't mix disinfectants with anything but water, according to the label directions. Even if a homemade cleaning cocktail doesn't cause a dangerous chemical reaction, it will probably decrease the disinfectant's efficacy.

- ✔ In case of an accident with the product, check the label for the first aid instructions, or call the Poison Control Center at 800-222-1222.

Providing a Healthy and Comfortable Environment

You can avoid many chicken health problems if you provide a safe, clean environment that's comfortable, from the chicken's perspective. These sections help remind you to keep your flock in mind as you create their little world.

Considering your chickens' coop

In order to give your flock a comfy environment, you need to start with the flock's coop. The coop should protect the chickens from predators, wind, rain, and hot sun, but it shouldn't be air-tight. Fresh air is very important to control moisture inside a chicken coop and prevent buildup of ammonia that results from the breakdown of droppings.

In cold climates, face the coop's doors and windows toward the midday sun for the warmest and driest orientation. In warm climates, orient the coop in the opposite direction, so openings don't face the sun during midday.

Provide enough space for everyone. Crowded chickens are more prone to disease and to injury from each other. See Table 5-2 for suggested space allowances for different types of chickens.

Table 5-2	Space Allowances for Chickens	
Type of Bird	*Square Feet Per Bird Inside*	*Square Feet Per Bird Outside*
Chicks: 0–4 weeks	½	--
Chicks: 4–8 weeks	1	--
Chicks: 8–12 weeks	2	--
Meat chickens in mobile pens, moved daily	--	1.5
Bantam chickens	2	6
Laying hens	3	8
Large-breed chickens	4	10

Creating comfy bedding

Chickens kept on a solid floor, such as a dirt or wood floor, should have some sort of absorbent bedding, to control moisture and serve as an insulating material in cold weather. Wood shavings are the most common bedding material for poultry, because they're absorbent, widely available, and relatively inexpensive. Many flock keepers are very creative at using the cheap, plentiful organic materials that are available where they live, and they've successfully raised poultry on all sorts of stuff, including sand, sawdust, shredded paper, leaves, or even coconut husk fiber. Availability and cost will probably drive your decision on which bedding to use for your flock.

Despite all the dire Internet warnings about the negative health effects of cedar shavings for poultry, we can't find any evidence that cedar shavings cause health problems for chickens. They're commonly used as poultry bedding wherever it is economical to do so.

Whatever you decide to use as bedding, keep the bedding dry, but not dusty. Neither mold nor dust is good for chickens to breathe long term, and constantly wet feet can turn into sore, infected feet. Stir the bedding every few days and move feeders and waterers to new locations so that wet areas don't develop. If they do, remove the wet bedding and add new, dry stuff.

The *deep litter method* has become popular among backyard flock keepers, especially lazy ones, for bedding chickens through the winter. Starting with at least 6 inches of bedding over a dirt floor, you periodically sprinkle new bedding on top. You occasionally stir the litter, but don't completely clean it out until spring. During six months, the layers may build up to several feet. The lower layer composts in place, breaking down through natural microbial action and generating heat, which is a welcome byproduct in cold weather. If deep litter is managed properly, it gives off little odor, and disease-causing organisms are cooked.

Handling outdoor runs

Most flock keepers like to see their chickens roaming outside, instead of being cooped up inside all the time. You can also manage outdoor runs in a healthful way, by allowing adequate space. We suggest space allowances for outdoor housing in Table 5-2.

The ground around pop holes or doors into a house often becomes muddy, so you can sprinkle sand, wood chips, or bedding over a muddy entrance, or put down a rubber mat, which you can easily pick up and periodically clean. You can't disinfect dirt, so chemical disinfection isn't an option for permanent, earth-floored outdoor runs, although they do benefit from frequent raking and twice yearly scraping-out and recharging with 3 to 4 inches of fresh, clean sand or wood chips.

If you're using a pasture, paddock, or tractor system to free-range your chickens, expect to move the birds regularly to prevent manure buildup and overgrazing. You may be moving chicken tractors every day or rotating paddocks weekly. More rapid rotation is better for disease control than allowing birds to remain in one place longer. After moving the chickens to a new location, rake the ground to break up droppings, and consider whether the area needs to be mowed. Filling in old dustbath holes to prevent them from becoming water-filled mosquito brooders or tripping hazards is also a good idea.

Managing adverse weather events

Preparation for seasonal changes in weather can prevent an uncomfortable spell of hot, cold, or wet weather from becoming a flock disaster. Consider your climate when you build your coop and choose breeds for your flock. Hot weather is hard on adult chickens, but with our help in these sections, they can cope. Keeping chicks warm in freezing weather is a challenge; adult chickens usually do just fine in the cold.

Dealing with hot weather

The living is easy for adult chickens when the temperature is between about 55 degrees F and 80 degrees F (10 degrees C and 27 degrees C), but temperatures higher than 80 degrees F (27 degrees C) reduce chickens' appetites, growth, egg production, and shell quality. The risk that birds may die from heat stress increases as the temperature rises above 90 degrees F (32 degrees C), especially for large breeds, meat chickens, and layers in full production. Chickens can acclimate to gradual increases in environmental temperatures, but sudden heat waves can be deadly.

You may have noticed that chickens don't sweat. Instead, they lose heat through combs, wattles, legs, and the nonfeathered areas under the wings, and by panting. Chickens also change their behavior to cope with the heat. We've seen many very creative strategies that backyard flock keepers use to cool their birds. Here are a few of those hot weather coping skills, along with flock keepers' strategies that take advantage of natural chicken behaviors:

✔ **Chickens avoid things that radiate heat, including each other, oven-like coops, and sunbaked earth.** Give your chickens plenty of space and shade. Provide them with a cool place to dustbathe. Insulate the coop roof and paint it white. Build the coop on stilts to provide a shady daytime resting spot underneath.

Keep the bedding in the coop to a minimum. Summer isn't the time to try the deep litter method (refer to the earlier section, "Creating comfy bedding," for information), because it generates heat. Bare dirt pens can become scorching hot, and long grass and weeds can block breezes; short grass is cooler.

✔ **During hot weather, chickens eat in early morning and late evening.** Feed the birds in early morning and again in the evening when the temperature drops. Digestion generates heat, so avoid feeding during the day. The best time to use cooling devices, such as fans, misters, soaker hoses, or frozen water bottles, is in the evening, to cool the chickens enough that they feel like eating dinner and breakfast.

✔ **In hot weather, chickens will drink more water if it's cool water.** A panting bird cools itself through evaporation of moisture from the throat and respiratory tract, so good hydration is critical. Always keep plenty of water in shady spots. Change the water often to keep it cool, or place frozen water bottles in waterers.

Don't handle or move your chickens in the hottest part of the day. If you must move them, do it at night when it's cooler.

Dealing with freezing weather

Compared to hot weather, managing freezing temperatures is a bit simpler for owners of adult chickens. As long as chickens are dry and protected from wind, they'll usually do just fine; they don't need a heated coop. Again, chickens have built-in environmental coping skills, which we list here, along with ways that flock keepers help their birds cope.

✔ **Chickens eat more in cold weather, because food provides energy for making body heat.** Always have a good-quality complete diet available. Feed *free-choice,* which means that you give the chickens as much as they're able to consume.

✔ **In cold weather, blood flow to heat-losing body parts, such as combs, wattles, and toes, is restricted.** Chickens are prone to frostbite in cold weather, especially chickens with large combs and wattles characteristic of certain breeds. (We discuss ways to recognize and deal with frostbitten body parts in Chapter 11.) Toes are more likely to become frostbitten if the floor of the coop or pen is wet, so keep the coop stocked with fresh, dry bedding. Ventilation is also important to keep the coop from becoming damp; don't close it up tight. Wintertime is a great time to use the deep litter method, because it generates heat.

✔ **In cold weather, chickens drink more if the water is warm.** Check waterers three to four times a day and replace frozen water with warm water, or use electric livestock water heaters. Several types are available at farm supply stores. Try not to let the birds go without water for more than a couple of hours. Chickens can't lick ice or get all the water they need by eating snow.

Chicks are a completely different story from adult chickens in wintertime; it's a challenge to keep them warm enough in cold weather. If you use heat lamps in brooders, hang two lamps and always have spare bulbs handy, in case one lamp stops working. Frequently check the brooder to ensure that the chicks are comfortable, not huddling, and that the heat source is working.

Electric heat lamps are the most commonly used source of heat for backyard flock brooders, but you must use them with extreme caution, because they can become fire hazards. Two styles of heat lamps are widely available:

✔ Lamps that are held in position with a clamp

✔ Lamps that are hung from the ceiling

The lamps with clamp attachments frighten us, so please don't use them. Clamp lamps are notorious for slipping, and we are aware of many tragic incidents involving baby livestock and this style of lamp. Purchase the type of lamp without a clamp that must be suspended from the ceiling. Hang the lamp with sturdy wire or chain, not flammable rope, and make sure the lamp can't touch anything around it. Put a smoke alarm in the brooder area, and check the alarm monthly to make sure it's working properly.

Disaster planning

Natural disasters, such as floods, hurricanes, and wildfires disrupt the lives of thousands of people (and their chickens!) every year. What makes the difference between extreme weather being deadly or simply inconvenient is your plan. Do you have one? Are you ready? If not, make sure you have a plan in case the worst happens.

In the United States, emergency management agencies at the federal, state, and local levels can provide guidance about the hazards in your area, and help you develop a plan, which would include these preparedness actions:

✔ **Be informed about the risks of weather emergencies in your area and about your community's emergency warning systems.** If you live in the United States, visit www.ready/gov/today to view information about hazards that can occur in your state. Your county's emergency management office can tell you about your community's emergency warning systems, which may include special sirens or radio broadcasts.

✔ **Consider options for evacuating your birds and for sheltering them in place.** Now, while the sky is blue and the wind is calm, find a place where your birds will be welcome if you decide to evacuate in an emergency, and plan a safe way to transport them.

If you intend to leave them behind, make a plan for providing a 48-hour food and water supply, at least. Identify each bird with a leg band or wing band, and record the identification number. Doing so may help you get them back if they're let loose during an emergency.

✔ **Put together an emergency supply kit.** Your kit may include carriers, material for temporary coops and pens, extra feeders and waterers, and a back-up source of water that doesn't depend on electricity.

✔ **Find an emergency contact.** This person should be someone who can check on the birds for you if you aren't able to do so.

Plan ahead. Your birds look to you to look out for them!

Chapter 6

Feeding the Flock Well

● ●

● ●

*F*eed is the major expense of raising chickens, unless of course, you built the chicken version of the Taj Mahal. Good nutrition means the difference between good health and production, or sorry-looking chickens who lay no eggs, so spending your money wisely makes sense.

In this chapter, we introduce you to the nutritional needs of chickens, which change during the stages of their lives. We also explain a bit about the way feed ingredients are made into diets for chickens and the variety of ways you can feed them. Finally, we provide some tips to preserve flock health and financial resources by storing chicken feed properly. You can also check out *Raising Chickens For Dummies* by Kimberly Willis and Rob Ludlow (John Wiley & Sons, Inc.).

Meeting Your Chickens' Nutritional Needs

Chickens must get protein, energy, vitamins, and minerals from their food. Different types of chickens need different nutrients, so different diets are fed depending on a chicken's age, sex, and occupation. In these sections, we outline what the different nutrients are and when your chickens need those nutrients during their lives.

Understanding nutrients

Nutrients are the substances in feed ingredients that sustain body maintenance, growth, production, and health. Nutrient needs are different, depending on the age, breed, and sex of the chicken. (Refer to the later section, "Recognizing nutritional needs of different life stages," for specifics.) A good diet for a chicken (or any animal, really) must have proper amounts of water, protein, carbohydrates, fats, vitamins, and minerals.

A chicken's body keeps the bird's nutritional priorities in order. Nutrients support basic maintenance body function first. After a chicken meets its basic needs, any extra nutrition can be used for performance, such as rapid growth in meat chickens, bountiful egg production in laying hens, or gorgeous plumage in show birds — or becoming a fat, bossy hen.

When the nutrients provided in the diet are less than optimal for a chicken's performance potential, the chicken will grow slower, lay fewer eggs, or not grow perfect, glossy feathers. If nutrients are so deficient that basic maintenance needs aren't met, chickens can become ill. We talk about diseases of nutritional deficiency in Chapter 11.

Water

Water is the most important nutrient for chickens, because lack of water can affect a chicken's health and performance quicker than a shortage of any other nutrient. A chicken consumes daily about twice the amount of water as feed, by weight.

Water helps the process of digestion by softening food in the *crop* (the pouch in the esophagus of chickens) and carrying food through the digestive tract. Most body processes and chemical reactions of life require water. In Chapter 5, we talk about the importance of water for birds to keep cool.

When you provide water to your chickens, make sure the water is clean, cool, and always available.

Protein

Chickens need *protein,* which is an important building block of body tissue. We wish it were that simple. Actually, chickens require enough of each of more than 20 amino acids, which comprise protein molecules. Chickens can make some of the amino acids inside their own bodies, but they can't make all of them, so they must get these essential animo acids from their diets.

Unfortunately, no single feed ingredient can provide all the required amino acids, so several sources of protein are used in a chicken feed, in order to cover all the bases. The main protein sources for commercial chicken feed are plant proteins, such as soybean meal and corn gluten meal, and animal proteins, such as meat meal or fish meal.

By looking at chickens' amino acid requirements, you can see that chickens aren't vegetarians by nature. Plant proteins are generally poor sources of some of the essential amino acids for chickens, but meat and other animal proteins — including chicken delicacies, such as crickets, earthworms, and fat, juicy caterpillars — are typically rich sources of those essential amino acids. Keeping chickens healthy on a purely vegetarian diet is possible, but nutritionists pay close attention to the plant protein sources in vegetarian chicken feed to make sure all the essential amino acids are in the diet.

Amino acid analysis is much more of a hassle and an expense than measuring the total protein content of feed, so feed manufacturers usually only list the protein content, rather than the levels of each amino acid, on the feed label. Doing so simplifies choosing a bag of commercial feed, because you usually only have the *crude protein analysis* (an estimate of the total protein content of the feed) to look at when making feed-buying decisions. When you buy a bag of chicken feed, you trust the nutritionists at the feed mill to balance the individual amino acids in the diet. If you mix your own chicken feed, however, balancing a ration for protein is more complicated that getting the total protein content right.

Carbohydrates

Carbohydrates are the major energy source in a chicken's diet. A chicken's digestive system breaks down carbohydrates into glucose, which is the sugar that the body's cells use for fuel. A variety of grains, such as corn, wheat, or oats, are the usual major sources of carbohydrates in chicken feed.

Fats

Like carbohydrates, *fats* are also important sources of energy. In fact, fats contain more than twice the energy as any other feed ingredient. Fat-soluble vitamins A, D, E, and K are absorbed into the body with the help of fat in the diet.

Fats consist of smaller pieces called fatty acids. Chickens' bodies can't make one type of fatty acid, *linoleic acid,* which is essential for good health and fertility, so the fat source in the diet must contain some linoleic acid. Fortunately, grains and processed plant fat sources, such as vegetable oil, contain plenty of linoleic acid.

Minerals

Chickens need *microminerals,* such as iron, copper, zinc, manganese, and iodine, for good health, but only in tiny amounts. Feed manufacturers add trace mineral mixes to chicken feed to supply microminerals. On the other hand, chickens require larger amounts of *macrominerals,* such as calcium, phosphorus, and salt. Ground oyster shell and limestone are good sources of calcium for chickens.

Avoid feeding dolomitic limestone (dolomite) to chickens as a calcium source, because the high magnesium content can cause a decrease in egg production.

Vitamins

Vitamins are a group of substances found naturally in foods in small quantities, which are necessary for normal body functions, growth, and reproduction. Chickens need more than a dozen different vitamins in their diet. Although some feed ingredients have a natural abundance of certain vitamins, feed manufacturers add a vitamin premix to commercial chicken feed to make sure enough of each of the vitamins is in the bag.

Recognizing nutritional needs of different life stages

Poultry diets are formulated for specific stages in a chicken's life and for the chicken's purpose. Check the feed bag label and tag of commercial poultry diets for nutrient levels, ingredients, and directions for use. Table 6-1 outlines a few critical nutrient needs at the different stages and purposes of a chicken's life.

Table 6-1	Nutrient Requirements of Different Ages and Types of Chickens			
Bird Type	**Age**	**Diet Type**	**Crude Protein (%)**	**Calcium (%)**
Broilers (meat-type chickens)	0–4 weeks	Starter/Grower	21–25	0.9–1.0
	4 weeks to slaughter	Finisher	19–23	0.8–1.0
Dual-purpose chicks and growing birds	0–18 weeks	Starter/Grower	18–19	0.8–1.0
Laying hens	> 18 weeks	Layer	14–16	3.0–3.4
Breeders	Adult	Layer/Breeder	14–16	2.7–3.5

The younger a chicken, the more protein it needs. Chicks need plenty of protein that provides all the essential amino acids for good health and growth. The protein needs of chicks decline as they mature. *Broilers* (meat-type chickens) are fed high protein diets to help them rapidly gain weight. Pullets destined to produce eggs are fed a lower protein diet that allows them to mature at a slower rate, to build a strong skeletal structure and healthy reproductive tract, without getting too fat.

Rations designed for baby chicks are called *starter* or *starter/grower* diets. Chicks raised in backyard flocks do well eating starter diets with 18 to 20 percent protein during their first month of life. In addition to chick starter diets, you may also find *grower, finisher,* or *developer* diets at your feed store or mill. These diets are intended for later stages of a young bird's life.

Egg-laying hens need large amounts of calcium for good eggshell development. Complete layer diets provide all the calcium laying hens need, but you can offer extra ground oyster shell or limestone for the hens to choose if they want it. Breeder chickens are expected to produce eggs that hatch healthy chicks. Layer diets are fortified with plenty of vitamins and minerals for producing good quality eggs, so layer diets are suitable for breeder chickens.

Don't feed layer diets to growing birds, or feed diets meant for growing birds to laying hens. The high calcium content of complete layer diets can cause growth problems, kidney damage, and death in growing birds. Laying hens fed lower-calcium grower diets will lay fewer eggs, and those eggs may be soft or malformed.

Comprehending Feeds and Feeding Programs

Feeds come in many different forms, such as mash, crumbles, or pellets. You can also find different feeding programs, such as whole grain, vegetarian, or organic feed. Your choices are bewildering. To help you make an informed choice, we simplify the nutrition lingo in the following sections.

You may be wondering about medicated feeds. You should intentionally and specifically use medicated feed only for certain disease prevention or control purposes, not blindly or routinely. Backyard flock keepers most commonly use medicated feed to control coccidiosis, a disease we talk about in Chapter 13, so for now, to keep it simple, we give this advice: if you don't know why you're considering buying or using a medicated feed, don't do it.

Spelling out the forms of feed

Chicken feed comes in several forms: whole grains, mash, pellets, or crumbles. Feed mills grind whole grains, add protein, vitamin, and mineral supplements and transform the mix into the various styles of processed poultry feed.

Whole grains

You can directly feed whole grains to chickens. Whole grains are a good source of energy and some vitamins, but they generally aren't good sources of protein or minerals. *Scratch,* for example, is usually a combination of two or three whole grains, such as wheat, oats, barley, sorghum, or corn.

A chicken must "chew" whole grains by grinding them in the muscular stomach, the *gizzard.* The presence of *grit* (small stones) in the gizzard helps the grinding process. Free-range chickens can usually find their own grit while roaming around, pecking in the dirt, but chickens confined to barns or cages need to be provided with a source of grit if they're fed whole grains. Chickens that regularly eat whole grains develop bigger gizzards than chickens fed small particles of feed, such as mash, because of the exercise from "chewing."

Research has shown that chickens who eat whole grains gain weight or produce eggs as well as or better than chickens fed finely ground feeds. An exception among commonly used grains is corn (maize). Chickens have difficulty eating whole kernels of corn, so feed manufacturers usually crack corn into pieces when it's included in whole grain chicken feeds.

Grain (such as scratch), by itself, isn't a complete and balanced diet for chickens at any stage of life. In order for a diet with whole grains to be complete, you must also feed your chickens a protein source, vitamins, and minerals along with the grains. Check out the next section for more information.

An advantage of whole grain diets is that they may be cheaper than complete processed diets, because less processing is involved. Whole grain diets can be very economical to feed if you grow your own grain, or if local supplies of grain are plentiful and inexpensive.

A disadvantage of whole grain diets is that chickens sort through whole grain mixes to pick and choose the stuff they like. If you don't provide the flock with enough food and room for every bird to have plenty of choice, the birds on the bottom on the pecking order, who are forced to eat last, get the less nutritious leftovers.

The result may be a flock with some fat, bossy hens, and some skinny hens at the bottom of flock society; both ends of the spectrum are an unhealthy state. You may be able to avoid this problem if you have plenty of feeder space for everyone to eat at the same time, and if you frequently offer fresh feed.

Mash

Grinding whole grains makes *mash.* A protein supplement, vitamins, and minerals are added to the ground grain to make a complete mash diet. Mash is commonly fed to confined layers and to chicks. Because the feed is finely ground, chickens don't need to "chew" it in the gizzard, and grit isn't necessary for digestion of mash.

Mash is easy for chicks to eat and digest, and it has other advantages, too. Because mash feed is finely ground, chickens can't pick through the feed to select certain ingredients, and the tiny particles of mash that inevitably get scattered around provide hours of foraging entertainment. The main disadvantages of mash are that it's very dry and dusty, and chickens waste quite a bit of it while scattering it around. You can add water to mash to make the feed less dusty and more palatable.

 If you have a problem with feather pecking in your flock, feeding a mash diet may help reduce that bad behavior, because it gives the hens something to peck at other than their neighbors.

Pellets

Pelleted feed is made by putting mash through a *pellet mill,* a machine that cooks the feed, usually with steam, and pushes it through holes in a metal plate to create feed pellets. To make a complete pelleted diet, feed manufacturers put a thoroughly mixed, finely ground combination of grains, protein sources, and a vitamin and mineral supplement into the pellet mill.

Pelleted feeds have several advantages over other forms of feed. The cooking process kills disease-causing organisms, such as *Salmonella* bacteria, that may be in the raw feed ingredients. Cooking also makes some nutrients in the feed easier to digest. Grit isn't required for chickens to digest this form of feed. Chickens tend to waste less feed if it's in pellet form, and they can't pick and choose ingredients — each pellet is a unit of complete nutrition.

Many flock owners worry that little bantam chickens may have difficulty eating pellets, which have the largest particle size of the processed feed types. The good news is that bantam chickens *can* eat pellets.

Some disadvantages are that pellet mills are expensive pieces of equipment, so pelleted feed tends to cost more that whole grain or mash diets. Pellets also are fast food — literally, not nutritionally — because chickens can quickly eat a pellet meal. Chickens naturally spend much of their day hunting for food, so chickens fed pellets may be bored chickens, looking for trouble.

Crumbles

Crumbles are simply crushed pellets. The smaller particles are easier for chicks to eat, so starter diets commonly come in the form of crumbles. Adult chickens tend to waste more crumbled feed than pelleted feed, because the particle size is smaller and they can scatter it more easily.

Eyeing the array of feeding programs

For generations, flock owners have raised and maintained healthy chickens by feeding all sorts of feedstuffs all sorts of ways. Perfectly adequate feeding programs range from the no-brainer approach of feeding a complete commercial diet, to programs that take a bit more thought and effort, such as mixing your own complete diet at home, or choice feeding, which we describe later.

The good news is no diet is best. You can choose a feeding program that works well for your particular situation and keeps your birds in good health. Your choice of a feeding program depends on how much interest, time, and money you have to devote to the program, your ideals and goals for your flock, and your access to feed ingredients.

Chickens have comfort foods. They generally stick to what they're familiar with, and they need time to learn about new foods and food choices. Don't try a new feed ingredient, feed form, or feeding program at a stressful time in the flock's life, such as during peak egg production, or when the flock is experiencing an illness.

The feeding programs most commonly used by owners of small flocks are complete commercial diets, complete home-mixed diets, and choice feeding. For each of these three programs, you can use conventional or organic ingredients, or rely on pasture for part of the flock's nutrition.

Complete commercial diet

The easiest way to feed a small flock of chickens is to buy a complete commercial diet from a feed store. Buying commercial feed is convenient and saves time. It may be the least expensive option for small flock owners, because it doesn't require bulk storage or mixing equipment. You don't need to have any special knowledge of nutrition in order to feed your birds well with a complete, commercial feed.

The feed bag label tells you what age and type of chicken the diet is designed for, and how to feed it. Most of these diets are designed to be fed *free-choice* — just keep the feeder full, all of the time.

Some flock owners have access to a feed mill that can mix a compete diet according to the customer's specifications. Custom mixes are often more expensive than commercial brands of chicken feed, and some mills require flock owners to purchase large quantities of feed at a time, which creates challenges for storage and preventing spoilage when you finally get all that custom-mixed feed home.

Complete home-mixed diet

For a variety of reasons, some flock owners mix their own feed at home. In some areas, using locally produced grains, discarded food, or food manufacturing byproducts, such as brewer's grains, as part of homemade diets for chickens may be more cost effective. Some flock keepers want to be precise about the ingredients that are fed to their chickens, or they want to use home-grown products, such as farmed insects or grains. Home-mixed diets may be the way to go for organic producers, because complete commercial organic feeds can be very expensive, especially if it must be shipped long distances.

The adventure of homemade chicken feed mixing isn't for the casual flock keeper, though. You need a solid knowledge of poultry nutrition to balance a ration properly and avoid nutritional deficiencies. Feeding unconventional feed ingredients does carry some risk because unexpected problems may happen, such as digestive upsets, toxicities, or spoilage. You need time, effort, and equipment to gather and store ingredients, grind grain, add supplements, and prepare mixes.

If you decide to go this route, you need to do a lot of reading. For starters, we recommend the book *Nutritional Requirements of Poultry* by the National Research Council. We also recommend that you find an experienced advisor for your homemade chicken feed project. Poultry nutritionists, feed mill operators, and extension agents can be good sources of advice. After you research and talk to an expert, you may want to try computer programs for feed formulation and least-cost calculation of feed ingredients that are available to balance your own homemade rations.

Choice feeding

The *choice feeding* option relies on the nutritional wisdom of chickens, the idea that chickens select a balanced diet if they're offered a variety of feed ingredients. *Nutritional wisdom* is a fairly well-documented phenomenon of chicken behavior. In several studies, chickens have demonstrated their ability to select a balanced diet from a buffet of goodies that meets their bodies' requirements for maintenance and production. Evidence suggests that, if you provide nutritious food options, you can trust your chickens to make nutritious food choices (well, maybe you can't trust the fat, bossy hen).

In a simple example of choice feeding, laying hens are provided three separate feeders, one containing a protein, vitamin, and mineral supplement, another feeder with whole grains (scratch), and a third with a calcium source of ground oyster shell or limestone. The hens eat cafeteria style from the feeders, and pick out the amounts of grain, supplement, and calcium source that they need to be healthy and productive.

Before adopting this method, we recommend that you do some additional reading about choice-feeding systems for chickens. A number of journal articles and online resources can give good explanations of the advantages and pitfalls.

Pasture

Pasture can provide some of a flock's nutritional needs and reduce the amount of purchased feed. A chicken's digestive system is designed to extract nutrients from seeds, insects, and worms, but not so much from leaves and twigs. Chickens aren't small cows, and they're unable to digest mature, tough grass and woody plants, but they can digest and extract some nutrients from young, tender grass and leafy plants.

Pastured poultry producers estimate that chickens can get 5 to 30 percent of their food from foraging on pasture. Summer pasture is often full of tasty insects and worms, which are packed with protein, fat, vitamins, and minerals. The best pasture isn't too tall, maybe two inches high, and has a variety of plants, including some protein-rich legumes, such as clover or alfalfa.

You can research ways to improve pasture and use those methods to cut your feed costs and please your flock. The American Pastured Poultry Producers Association (APPPA) and other sustainable agriculture organizations provide online resources. Check out the APPPA website at www.apppa.org. Agriculture departments at universities and extension agents are also good sources of information about pasture management.

Organic feed

Under U.S. Department of Agriculture National Organic Program rules, certified organic poultry must be fed certified organic feed. The rules are complicated, but in a nutshell, organic feed ingredients are produced without synthetic pesticides or fertilizers. Also, organic feed can't contain supplements or additives that are prohibited by the National Organic Program List of Allowed and Prohibited Substances, which names substances that are natural as well as synthetic.

Organic feed can be processed and presented to chickens in any of the feed forms or feeding programs we mention in this chapter. A big challenge of keeping poultry healthy with organic feed is providing enough *methionine* (an essential amino acid), because only a few allowable sources of methionine are available.

For more information about the National Organic Program visit the USDA Agricultural Marketing Service website (www.ams.usda.gov/nop/). Many other countries have organic programs with different sets of rules that describe how organic feed must be produced.

Keeping Feed Fresh

Regardless of how you choose to feed your birds, storing it properly is important so that it keeps its nutritional value. Nutrients, especially vitamins, deteriorate over time.

The good ol' days of homemade chicken feed

Have you ever wondered how flock keepers fed their chickens in the days before the convenience of nutritionally complete and balanced, bagged chicken feed? Some lucky chickens ate four home-cooked meals a day, from a menu that read like one from a gourmet health-food restaurant.

In 1888, Mr. I. K. Felch, well-known breeder of thoroughbred fowl and author of the book *Poultry Culture,* recommended a bill of fare for young chickens with different dishes for each day of the week. Here is the menu for Wednesdays:

"Breakfast: Fish chowder made palatable with salt and pepper, boiled potatoes, and thickened with cornmeal and shorts." (*Shorts* are the fine particles left over from milling wheat flour.)

Ten o'clock: Oats and wheat, and all the steamed clover or green chopped oats they would eat.

Dinner: Cracked corn and balance of the chowder if not wholly disposed of at the morning meal.

Supper: Cracked corn and barley."

We wish we could have been at the table for Mr. Felch's Friday meat soup with cornbread and milk!

To provide high-quality feed, follow these tips:

✔ **Store feed in a clean, cool, dry, rodent-proof area.** Your chickens can get sick from feed contaminated by animal droppings, and mold from a dirty, damp, pest-infested storage space. High temperatures hasten the deterioration of nutrients in the feed.

✔ **Keep the feed in its original bag inside a metal garbage can with a tight-fitting lid.** Metal garbage cans are excellent for keeping rodents out of bagged feed, but direct contact of the feed with the metal can cause chemical reactions that rapidly break down vitamins and fats, so that's why you use the original bag.

✔ **If the metal garbage can tip doesn't work for your situation and you must stack feed sacks in a room, store the sacks up off the floor on wood or plastic pallets.** Doing so prevents the bottom of the sacks from becoming damp. Damp food rapidly spoils and becomes moldy, and some types of spoilage bacteria and mold growth can make chickens sick.

✔ **To prevent feeders from becoming caked with old, moldy feed, let the birds clean up (run out of their feed) at least once a week, or empty the feeders.** Being out of feed for an hour or two in the afternoon won't hurt them.

✔ **Don't store feed for more than a month in the summer, or more than two months in the winter.** Proteins, fats, and vitamins deteriorate with time in storage and lose their nutritional quality.

✔ **If you moisten mash with water before you feed it, make it up fresh just before using it, and get rid of the uneaten wet mash at the end of the day.** The high moisture content of wet mash encourages bacteria to grow and the food spoils rapidly.

✔ **If the feed gets wet or looks moldy, don't feed it to the chickens.** We don't think it's worth the risk of illness caused by mold toxins or botulism (see Chapter 11 for more detail on these accidents of feed management).

Part II
Recognizing Signs of Chicken Illness

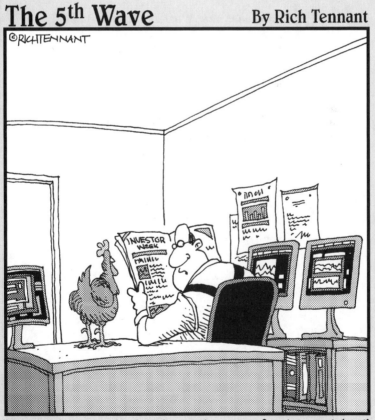

The 5th Wave   By Rich Tennant

©RICHTENNANT

"Invest in corn derivatives? Are you feeling alright?"

In this part...

"My chicken is sick. What can it be?" That's the question that we help you answer in Part II, which is a troubleshooting manual for chicken health problems commonly seen in backyard flocks. Sharpen your diagnostic skills using the techniques of flock inspection and physical examination we present in Chapter 7. Chapter 8 focuses on the glaring signs of health problems in adult chickens, and Chapter 9 covers signs of problems in chicks and growing birds. Chapter 10 tackles the challenging cases of subtle illness or sudden death, which may be difficult to diagnose.

Chapter 7

Inspecting the Flock and Examining the Sick Chicken

We hope that you've been fortunate, and you've never had a sick chicken in your flock. If that's the case, you're more than likely doing a good job with biosecurity and with keeping the flock clean, comfortable, and fed well. Even with the best of care, though, illness will occur in a flock sooner or later. You don't have complete control over your birds' environment, and except for the mythical phoenix, no bird lives forever.

When the inevitable occurs, can you quickly recognize the sick chicken? If you spend daily quality time with your birds, spotting the one that is under the weather will be easier. In this chapter, we describe how to make the most of that quality time. That's just the first step to a diagnosis, though, because next you need to closely examine a sick bird and take a holistic look at the flock, in order to zero in on the problem. We help you perform a thorough physical examination, step by step. At the end of this chapter, we provide a checklist to help you make sure you've gathered as many clues as possible. Then, you can give your chicken health advisor the best shot at making a correct diagnosis.

Tuning in to Your Flock

Flock keepers who really know their birds are not only aware of how much the birds usually eat and drink in a day, but they're also tuned in to their normal activities, sounds, and smells. They sense immediately when something is amiss in the behavior of the flock. You can become tuned in to your flock by spending daily quality time with your birds, by observing the flock from a distance, and by taking notes on activities and events in the flock.

Inspecting the flock

One of the joys of keeping chickens is the peaceful daily visit to the coop to watch the chickens being chickens. At the end of a long day, you probably de-stress by strolling with the hens in the yard and throwing them a little scratch, or by just sitting and observing them interacting with their world and with each other. That daily (or more often) observation is restful for you, and it's also good for the flock.

Chickens view people as predators, until proven otherwise. You can prove yourself safe in your chickens' eyes and reduce fear in the flock through regular, positive interactions with them. Predators act unpredictably; they stare, stalk, move suddenly, and pounce. Safe people behave predictably, the same way every day; they avoid prolonged eye contact, move casually and slowly, and bring good things to eat. Research shows that flocks of chickens who interact frequently with people in a positive way suffer less stress, fear, illness, and injury; they also grow faster, and produce more eggs.

At a regular time each day, spend at least a few minutes of quality time with your flock. Unless you have a large number of chickens, do a head count and quickly make a mental note of each chicken's behavior. Slowly walk among them. Touch a bird only if you're invited (a bird jumping up on your lap or your shoulder is an obvious invitation). Throw a few food treats. Does every bird run for the treats you tossed?

Use your senses as you stroll through the flock. Do you feel flies or mosquitos pestering you? Do you feel wet bedding? Can you see any watery droppings under the perches? Do you hear any unusual sounds, such as coughing, sneezing or snicking? (A sneezing chicken makes a *snick* sound.) Do you smell anything unusual? Moldy or spoiled feed may have a distinctive bad odor. Diarrhea or discharge from wounds or runny eyes and nostrils smell even worse. Investigate unusual sounds or smells and try to find their sources.

Spying on the flock: Observing chickens from a distance

Many critters like to eat chickens, and chickens instinctively know they're on the menu. Predators are naturally lazy; they would rather not work hard for a meal, so they usually focus on prey that's easily caught — the animal that looks less alert and slower than the others in the group. A chicken's best interest is to appear to be bright-eyed, alert, and in vigorous good health at all times. This instinct for self-preservation causes sick chickens to pretend to be well, until they're so sick that they can't put on the act anymore. The act is called *masking behavior.*

To look behind the mask, try to observe the flock when the birds don't know you're looking at them. The birds will be less alert and less likely to be putting on the "I'm healthy and fast; you can't catch me" act if they don't think they're being watched. Start and end your flock visits by observing them from a distance for a minute or two. Are all of the birds walking normally? Is any bird separated from the rest of the flock? Which birds are eating and drinking? Is any bird breathing hard or with an open mouth?

A chicken who looks ill to you is probably *very sick,* maybe for a while now, because the bird has been masking the illness, pretending everything was okay. Don't handle that chicken much, because that bird is already in distress, and rough handling can be the straw that breaks the camel's back. Treat the sick chicken quickly and gently. Read on for suggestions about handling and restraint.

Measuring performance and writing it down

If you ask for help with a chicken health problem, your chicken health advisor will want to know your flock's stats. (See Chapter 15 for tips on finding a chicken health advisor.) Keep track of the following information so you're prepared when your chicken health advisor asks you questions about your sick birds:

- ✔ **Age of the flock and stage of production:** How old are the birds? How many weeks have the hens been laying (or been *in lay*)?

- ✔ **Daily egg production:** How many eggs per day does the flock usually lay? Is egg production going up or down lately?

- ✔ **Date of last molt:** When did the flock last go through a molt? (You can read more about molting feathers in Chapter 2.)

✔ **Daily feed and water consumption:** How much does the flock usually eat and drink in a day? Is food and water consumption going up or down? You may measure feed and water in pounds and gallons, or in the number of scoops and jugs, or how often you fill the feeder or waterer.

You may have a difficult time answering these questions, especially if you didn't write down important dates and amounts. Having that information jotted down somewhere can be helpful to you if you need to investigate a sick chicken and ask for help. Your record-keeping system can be as simple as a paper coop notebook or as elaborate as an electronic database. (There should be an app for that!) Refer to the later section, "Recording Your Findings," for what to record and how.

Recognizing the General Signs of Illness

Before you can help a sick chicken, you need to know how to identify a sick chicken. Figure 7-1 shows a droopy chicken, exhibiting several signs of illness. Here's how a droopy chicken looks and acts:

✔ The head is hanging down and the eyes are slightly or completely closed. (Perhaps a headache?)

✔ The bird is huddled or crouching.

✔ Feathers are ruffled, especially the feathers on the back of the neck. The bird may look *puffed up.*

✔ The bird is reluctant to stand or move when you approach.

✔ The bird sits with his lower legs dropped to the ground, a posture called *hock sitting.*

✔ The bird separates itself from the rest of the flock.

✔ The bird eats or drinks less, or not at all.

Seeing one or more of these signs of illness tells you that you have a sick chicken on your hands. Each of the signs can range from very mild to very severe.

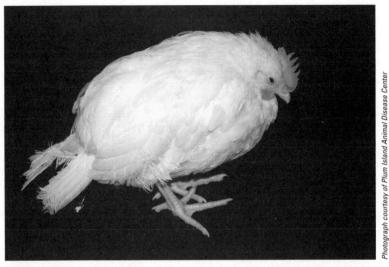

Figure 7-1: A droopy chicken.

If you spot one or more of these signs, are you ready to get on the phone with your vet to ask for a diagnosis, or post a request for a treatment plan from your online flock-keeper friends? Not yet. These signs only tell you something is wrong, but they don't tell you *what*. If you ask for advice at this point, you're likely to receive more questions than answers. The next step is to do a more detailed investigation of the chicken and the rest of the flock in order to find the clues that may lead you to a diagnosis.

Don't give any drugs based only on the general signs of illness we list in the preceding section. These signs aren't specific enough to give you a diagnosis and understand how to appropriately treat the flock. Collect more information and seek advice before you administer medication. In the best-case scenario, giving the wrong drug wastes money; at worst, the wrong drug can be harmful to your chickens or to people, if they eat eggs or meat from the treated birds.

Zeroing In on the Problem: The Physical Examination

After you recognize the sick chicken, you need to do a physical examination to collect more clues about the problem. The steps of a physical exam are

1. Catch and hold the chicken.

2. **Examine the head.**

3. **Evaluate the respiratory system and body condition.**

4. **Look at the skin and feathers.**

5. **Look at the wings, legs, and feet.**

6. **Examine the abdomen and vent.**

The following sections provide more detail about each of these steps.

 A chicken physical exam rarely includes taking the temperature or pulse. The body temperature varies widely in a chicken, usually between 105 and 107 degrees Fahrenheit (40.6 and 41.7 degrees Celsius), depending on when the bird has eaten, the chicken's breed and sex, the temperature of the environment, and other factors. A single thermometer reading doesn't tell you much, so we don't think that temperature-taking is worth the stress on the chicken (or you). A chicken's heart rate is very fast, as much as 400 beats per minute, so the pulse is almost impossible to feel and count.

Catching and holding the sick chicken

The first step in examining your sick chicken is catching it and then holding it so you can start the examination. Because heat stress is often deadly for sick chickens, you want to hold off on catching and holding a sick chicken until a cooler part of the day, if possible. If it's an emergency and you must examine a sick chicken during the hottest part of the day, do it quickly and do it in a cool spot, such as in the shade or in an air-conditioned room. (In Chapter 5, we talk about how healthy chickens have a difficult time dealing with hot weather.)

Here are three options for catching your patient, which we list from the easiest to the one that involves the most exercise for both the flock keeper and chicken.

- ✔ **Easy method**: Wait until dark to catch and examine a suspect sick chicken. Chickens have poor nighttime vision and don't move around much in the dark. In dim light, you can simply lift the bird off a perch with little fuss and carry the bird into a well-lit place for the exam.

- ✔ **Tame chicken method**: You may not have the luxury of waiting until dark to catch a chicken, but that's okay, because picking up an alert chicken who is in a decent mood isn't a huge challenge. Chickens who are used to being around people are usually very easy to catch and hold. Shoo them gently into the corner of the coop or pen, and catch your suspect bird by reaching both of your hands over her back and holding the wings down to restrain her. Then, move one of your hands down the front of the bird and under the abdomen and pick her up. You can carry her that way: one hand on her back and the other under her belly with your fingers between the legs. If you tuck her head loosely under your arm, she'll feel safer and be calmer.

✔ **Wild chicken method:** You may be in for a backyard rodeo if the chicken you're trying to catch isn't used to people or has a bad temper. You can catch ill-mannered roosters or wild hens with a net or a *poultry hook,* which is a pole about 4 feet long with a handle on one end and a hook on the other. You catch a chicken with the pole by using the hooked end to snag a leg anywhere above the foot, and then moving up quickly to grab the bird. You can purchase nets and poultry hooks from poultry supply companies.

Although a healthy chicken can be carried upside down by the legs without physical harm, a bird is scared by being handled that way. *Don't* carry a sick chicken by the legs. It's too stressful, and the bird can regurgitate food from the crop and inhale it, which can be fatal.

Examining the head

The second step of the sick bird examination is checking the bird's head. The less you restrain the bird, the better when you examine the head area. You don't need to grab the chicken tightly or hold the chicken's head still to get a good look. Let the chicken stand or sit on a flat, level surface, like a table or workbench, where you don't need to bend over. Look for these clues of chicken health problems:

✔ Swelling of the comb, eyelids, face, or wattles.

✔ Scabs anywhere on the head.

✔ An eye that is cloudy, goopy, or squinting. You also want to look for an irregularly shaped pupil. The pupil should be round and black.

✔ Crusty or runny nostrils.

✔ A beak that looks twisted to the side or has cracks. The upper and lower beaks should meet at the tips.

Evaluating the respiratory system and overall body condition

During your examination of the bird's head, the chicken hopefully settled down a little from being caught and carried. Now that the chicken is standing or sitting relaxed on the table, with only light restraint from you, take a look at how the bird is breathing.

You can hardly notice normal breathing. A chicken with respiratory problems breathes with an open mouth, and the tail may bob up and down with each breath. If the problem is in the upper part of the respiratory system, such as in the nostrils or windpipe, breathing may become easier as the bird relaxes. If the problem is in the lower part of the respiratory system, such as in the lungs or air sacs, open-mouth breathing and tail bobbing will continue even after the bird relaxes. (See Chapter 2 for a description of chicken respiratory system.)

Next, feel the *keel* (breastbone) to get an overall picture of body condition, to determine whether the chicken is thin or fat. Place your palm over the chest and keel of the bird. The keel sticks out from the bird's chest and is surrounded on each side by the breast muscles. You can score the body condition of your bird by the way the keel and breast muscles feel. See Table 7-1 for a description of the scoring system and Figure 7-2 for a visual.

Table 7-1	Chicken Body Condition Scoring System
Score	*Characteristics*
0	The edge of the keel is rough, sharp, and prominent. Very little breast muscle can be felt, and the breast on either side of the keel feels hollow or concave. This bird is very thin.
1	The keel is prominent, but doesn't feel sharp. There is some breast muscle, and the breast on either side of the keel feels flat. This bird is thin.
2	The keel is less prominent, and the edge is smoother. The breast muscle is well developed. The breast on either side of the keel is rounded or convex. This bird is in good condition.
3	The keel feels smooth and not very prominent. Feeling the edge of the keel may be difficult through the plump, rounded breast muscles. This is a fat bird.

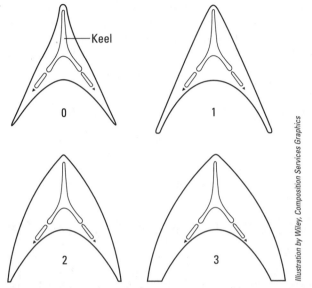

Keel

0

1

2

3

Illustration by Wiley, Composition Services Graphics

Figure 7-2: Diagrams of the keel and breast muscles for body condition scores 0-3.

Looking at skin and feathers

To continue your examination, lift up the feathers to look at the chicken's skin. Check for external parasites. Do you see any scurrying specks or walking dandruff? Look at the shafts of the feathers. White clumps on the feather shafts may be lice eggs; see Chapter 13 for a visual.

Go over the whole bird, stroking the feathers backward, to find areas of feather loss or skin that is reddened, lumpy, scabby, torn, or bruised. The color of a bruise can tell you the age of the injury. A bruise that just happened is red, and changes from purple, to green, to yellow, as it heals over three to five days.

Looking at wings, legs, and feet

For the first part of this step of the exam, the chicken should still be standing or sitting on the table. You can hold her lightly, restraining her only enough to prevent her from jumping off the table. Look at the bird's posture. Does she put weight on both legs evenly? Are both wings tucked up on her back, or does one of the wings droop? A bird that is reluctant or unable to put weight on a leg or tuck up a wing may be in pain or have nerve damage.

In the next part of this step, lay the chicken down on her side to examine more closely one wing, both legs, and both feet. Turn her over to the other side to examine the other wing. The chicken will usually lie quietly if you drape a light cloth, such as a dish towel, over her head.

Extend each wing to look for swelling, cuts, or bruising. The chicken shouldn't mind having her wings extended; if she struggles when you extend a wing, the reaction may be a sign of pain. Check the skin of the legs and feet. The scales should be smooth and straight. Upturned or rough leg scales can be a sign of mite infestation. Pay close attention to the bottoms of the feet; look for scratches, scabs, sores, or swellings.

Checking the abdomen and vent

In the last step of the examination, with the bird lying on her side, you can pick up the tail feathers to examine the vent area. Check for reddened, swollen, or torn skin and missing feathers. Look for blood coming from the vent or tissue protruding from it.

Gently feel the bird's abdomen; the chicken shouldn't mind you doing so, unless she is in pain. A hen who is laying eggs has a wide, moist vent and a soft, doughy, enlarged abdomen. A firm abdomen and a small, puckered, dry vent are signs that a hen isn't currently laying eggs.

A bird with diarrhea often has soiled feathers in the vent area. Loose, pasty white or yellow droppings may be stuck to reddened or swollen skin around the vent.

Recording Your Findings

From your physical examination, you have quite a bit of information to start figuring out the cause of the problem. You can use Table 7-2 to organize your findings and make communicating easier with your chicken health advisor. Circle your findings from each part of the exam. When you talk to your chicken health advisor, you can go down the list and avoid forgetting the important details gathered from your exam.

Table 7-2	Physical Examination Findings
Vital Sign or Body Part	*Potential Findings*
Egg production (hen)	Going up, going down, not laying
Feed and water consumption	Going up, going down, not eating/drinking
Head	Discharge, swelling, scabs, abnormal shape
Breathing at rest	Open-mouth, tail bobbing
Body condition	0, 1, 2, 3
Skin	Parasites, injury, lumps, scabs, abnormal color
Missing feathers	Head, neck, back, breast, wing, tail, abdomen, vent
Wings, legs, and feet	Signs of pain or weakness, rough leg scales, injury, sores, swelling
Abdomen	Soft, firm, enlarged, signs of pain
Vent	Pasty, injury, protruding tissue

The history of the sick bird and the rest of the flock is also important information, so share the notes from your coop notebook with your advisor, including the bird's age, where the bird came from, and how long the bird has been in the flock. Other key questions include how many other birds are sick and whether any birds have died recently. Be prepared to discuss how you feed, water, and house your flock.

Chapter 8

Troubleshooting Common Illnesses in Adult Chickens

* *

In This Chapter

▶ Relating to chicken head colds and stomach bugs

▶ Dealing with mishaps of the egg-laying plumbing

▶ Looking deep into your chicken's eyes and seeing something not quite right

▶ Determining whether feather loss isn't just a bad plumage day

▶ Limiting the confusion for a dizzy chicken

▶ Puzzling over limping hens and swollen feet

* *

"*W*hat causes that?" The purpose of this chapter is to help you answer that question by troubleshooting possible causes for the problem you're having with an adult chicken (say, older than 5 months old). (If you're concerned about a problem in a chick, check Chapter 9.) The signs of chicken illnesses that we discuss in this chapter are the ones that jump up and down at you, waving a red flag. You can commonly see these alarming signs in backyard flocks.

Each of the problems we discuss in this chapter has more than one possible cause, so we provide some diagnostic suggestions to help you get to the bottom of it. Veterinary diagnostic laboratories and avian veterinarians have the resources to help. To make the poor chicken feel a little better while you're waiting for a diagnosis (or if you're unable to get a diagnosis), we offer general supportive care advice for each problem. We don't get too deep into each of the diseases mentioned in this chapter; you can find more detailed information about the specific diseases in Chapters 11–14.

Sneezing and Coughing: Chicken Head Colds

Typical signs include sneezing, wheezing, coughing, and runny nose and eyes. The miserable patient also suffers fatigue and loss of appetite. You may prescribe chicken soup, but that somehow seems . . . *wrong*, when the patient is a chicken. For a human or a chicken, the signs of an upper respiratory infection are similar, but the causes are very different. With the exception of a few strains of avian influenza, you can't catch a cold from your chicken, and vice versa. We list infections of adult chickens in Table 8-1 that all cause sneezing, coughing, runny eyes, and runny nostrils. You can find in-depth information on each of these diseases in Chapter 12. If you're looking for causes of respiratory illness in chicks and growing birds, check Chapter 9.

Table 8-1 Causes of Respiratory Illness in Adult Chickens

Disease	Occurrence in Backyard Flocks	Distinctive Signs of Illness	Average Mortality Rate
Mycoplasmosis	Common	Foamy eye discharge, more common in winter, roosters usually show more severe signs	Usually none
Infectious coryza	Common	Swollen face or wattles, gunky eyes, foul odor, more common summer and fall	5–20 percent
Infectious bronchitis	Common	Decreased egg production	Usually none
Newcastle disease	Mild strains are common. Highly deadly strains are absent from chickens in the United States.	May also cause diarrhea, staggering, paralysis, sudden death	5–99 percent

Disease	Occurrence in Backyard Flocks	Distinctive Signs of Illness	Average Mortality Rate
Fowl cholera (chronic form)	Not so common	Swollen face, gunky eyes, rattling or difficulty breathing, more common in late summer	0–20 percent
Infectious laryngotracheitis (ILT)	Not so common	Gasping, coughing up bloody mucous, dried blood around nostrils and lower beak	10–20 percent
Avian influenza	Rare (Deadly strains are absent from chickens in the United States)	Droopy birds, rattling breathing sounds, diarrhea, sudden death	5–99 percent

Chicken respiratory infections can be so mild they're unnoticeable, or so severe that most of the flock dies in a short period of time. In severe cases, affected chickens may make rattling breathing sounds, gasp for air, or sling mucous from the mouth while shaking their heads. Sometimes a chicken's face will swell, especially around the eyes, cheeks, or wattles. The comb may turn a bluish color. The disease's severity depends on the organism strain and on the flock's overall health at the time the disease strikes.

Chicken respiratory infections are usually spread by direct contact between infected and uninfected chickens, but stuff that infected chickens have sneezed or coughed on, such as transport coops or clothing, can carry the infectious organisms from place to place, too. An infected hen can transmit mycoplasmosis through her eggs to her chicks.

Preventing respiratory illness from invading your flock and having a major impact is a matter of good biosecurity and flock management; see Chapters 4 and 5 for tips. The infections in Table 8-1 are all highly contagious, so attention to *biosecurity* (things you do routinely to keep infectious diseases out of your flock) can help you avoid bringing respiratory infections home to your chickens. If an infection should happen to get through your defenses, a clean, comfortable, and well-fed flock is less likely to experience severe disease.

Diagnosing chicken respiratory illness

You can guess, but you won't be able to tell for certain which disease is causing your chickens' woes, unless you have laboratory tests performed. Veterinary diagnostic laboratories and veterinarians who treat poultry can help you; see Chapter 15 for tips on working with a chicken health advisor to make a specific diagnosis.

Although diagnostic tests will cost you some money, getting to the bottom of the problem may be worth the expense, because a diagnosis allows you to

✔ **Know whether your birds are likely to be contagious and spread the infection to other birds.** This concern is especially important if you breed and sell birds or take birds to shows. Chickens can recover from the infections in Table 8-1 and appear healthy, but carry and spread the disease to other chickens, possibly for the rest of their lives.

✔ **Choose a medication that is likely to work.** Antibiotics are helpful to control the signs of some infections, but not others. Certain antibiotics kill certain organisms, but have no effect on others. If you get a diagnosis, you'll be able to use the appropriate drug; if not, you may have to play antibiotic roulette and hope you've picked the right one — or spin again.

✔ **Know whether a vaccine can help you control the problem.** Vaccines are available that help control several respiratory infections, including infectious coryza, mycoplasmosis, and infectious laryngotracheitis. For a number of reasons which we discuss in Chapter 16, we don't recommend using a vaccine for chicken disease control unless you know your flock is infected or likely to become infected.

Getting a diagnosis may bring more attention to your flock than you expected. In the United States, some or all the diseases listed in Table 8-1 are *reportable* in most states, meaning that laboratories and veterinarians are required by law to report the presence of the disease in your flock to the state veterinarian's office. What officials do with the report varies from state to state. In some places, your flock may be placed under quarantine, and you'll be required to prove that the infection has been cleaned up before birds can leave your place alive.

To see which chicken diseases are reportable where you live in the United States, look up your state at www.biosecuritycenter. org/reportDisease.php.

Giving supportive care for chicken respiratory illness

The four possible outcomes to chicken respiratory illness are as follows:

- ✔ Complete recovery, typically within two to four weeks
- ✔ The chicken recovers, but becomes a long-term carrier of the infection
- ✔ Chronic (long-term) illness
- ✔ Death

The chicken cold that never goes away (or comes back again and again) is probably *chronic respiratory disease* (CRD), caused by mycoplasmosis. For more details about CRD, see Chapter 12.

Chicken respiratory diseases are highly contagious. They cause a lot of trouble year after year in infected flocks, which are constant threats to uninfected flocks. You can't tell which recovered birds are carriers of infection without testing. Antibiotics make affected chickens feel better and may save a few that would have died without treatment, but antibiotics don't cure the infection in carrier birds or eliminate the disease from the flock.

If you discover respiratory illness in your flock, you're faced with a very difficult decision: *culling, depopulating,* or controlling. Your three choices aren't easy:

- ✔ Cull (another word for euthanize) affected birds to prevent spread of the disease in the flock.
- ✔ Depopulate the flock (euthanize all birds) to eliminate the infection. Then, clean up and start over.
- ✔ Live with the infection, using vaccination or medication to control illness.

If you decide to live with the problem, here are the do-it-yourself steps for treating mild respiratory illness affecting a small proportion of the flock:

1. **Self-impose a quarantine on your flock.**

   Don't move birds in or out.

2. **Isolate affected birds in a hospital pen and provide TLC.**

   We describe good nursing care in Chapter 17. Keep the hospital pen super-clean. Avoid dust and dirty bedding, which irritate sore lungs and sinuses.

3. **Use an antibiotic that is labeled for chicken respiratory illness, according to label directions.**

   Products with erythromycin, tetracycline, or tylosin are good first-line antibiotic choices that are available at many feed stores.

Consult your veterinarian if you want to treat laying hens, because no antibiotic is approved for use by U.S. flock keepers for laying hens. We discuss antibiotic use in more detail in Chapter 16.

Dealing with the Runs: Diarrhea in Adult Chickens

Some loose droppings are normal for chickens. Several times a day, a chicken passes sticky, smelly brown cecal poops that you may mistake for diarrhea. (See Chapter 2 for more on chicken digestive anatomy.) Droppings that look like cecal poops should make up no more than one-third of the droppings you see in the coop under the perches in the morning.

Flock keepers usually recognize diarrhea in a flock of chickens when they see hens with dirty vents or stained eggs. Chickens with diarrhea usually have matted feathers around the vent, which is a helpful indicator to you about which bird has the problem. A normal hen isn't perfectly clean back there, but in a hen with a problem, the feathers and the vent area are heavily pasted with dried yellowish poop, and the vent area may be red and sore-looking. Figure 8-1 shows a chicken with diarrhea and her dirty vent.

What does the color or consistency of droppings tell you about a chicken's health? Nothing specific. You can see a huge range of colors and consistencies in normal and abnormal chicken droppings. We haven't found that color or consistency predicts the fortune (or cause) of a chicken with diarrhea, so we won't ask you to "read" the droppings, either.

So many things can cause adult birds to have diarrhea, that we can't list them all here. Table 8-2 contains some of the most famous offenders. Flock keepers often think of intestinal worms as prime suspects, and intestinal parasites do cause a lot of trouble in young birds, but they're overrated as causes of diarrhea in adult chickens.

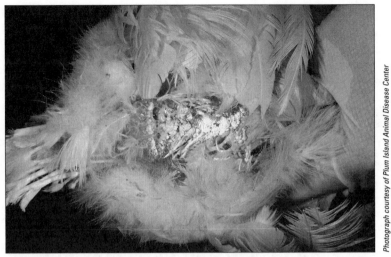

Photograph courtesy of Plum Island Animal Disease Center

Figure 8-1: A dirty vent of a chicken with diarrhea.

Table 8-2   Some Causes of Diarrhea in Adult Chickens

Type of Disease	Common Causes	Not-So-Common Causes	Rare Causes
Accidents of flock management (see Chapter 11)	Heat stress Vent prolapse	Excess salt in the diet Hardware disease Mold toxins in feed Raw soybean meal	Toxic plants
Bacteria or viruses (see Chapter 12)	Colibacillosis Lymphoid leukosis Marek's disease	Avian intestinal spirochetosis Avian tuberculosis Fowl cholera Infectious coryza	Avian influenza Newcastle disease
Parasites (see Chapter 13)	Coccidiosis	Heavy infections with threadworms	Blackhead

Diagnosing diarrhea in adult chickens

Even poultry veterinarians and diagnostic laboratories are stumped about the cause of chicken diarrhea. Fecal exams will probably show a few intestinal worm eggs and coccidia, but that's normal for adult free-range chickens. X-rays may show problems in the abdomen, such as *hardware disease* or *egg peritonitis,* diseases which have miserably low chances for recovery. The hard truth is that the most useful test for flock diarrhea is a postmortem exam of affected birds by a veterinary pathologist, but we realize that's not a helpful suggestion for dealing with the illness of a family pet.

For intestinal problems, a very fresh dead bird can provide the most useful information. In fact, it may be best to have sick birds euthanized at the laboratory and examined immediately. Call the laboratory ahead of time to make arrangements. See Chapter 15 for tips on submitting a bird for postmortem examination at a diagnostic laboratory.

Giving supportive care for an adult chicken with diarrhea

The following are do-it-yourself tips for dealing with adult chicken diarrhea while you're waiting for a diagnosis (or if you're unable to get one). You'll know within a week if your efforts are paying off. If the bird continues to decline despite your care, something sinister is going on; consider euthanasia and a postmortem. (See Chapters 15 and 18 for more information.)

- ✔ **If a small proportion of the flock is affected, isolate the sick birds in a hospital pen and provide good nursing care.** Birds with dirty vents may need to be housed individually in separate cages, because other birds like to peck at the raw area. If most of the flock is affected, leave the flock where it is and treat the whole flock. (See Chapter 17 for TLC tips.)

- ✔ **Check the flock's environment.** Is it clean and comfortable? Take steps to cool heat-stressed birds or dry out a wet pen. Clean waterers and provide fresh, clean water. Examine the diet. Did you feed something new? Check for moldy or spoiled feed. If you have any suspicions about the feed, change it, preferably to a fresh batch of a well-known brand of commercial layer feed.

- ✔ **Be on the lookout for vent prolapse.** If you see pink tissue protruding from the vent, read on for information about *blow-outs,* which can be the cause or the result of diarrhea/dirty vents.

- ✔ **Add two tablespoons of vinegar to each gallon of drinking water.** Vinegar is a "Why not?" remedy. Some evidence suggests that organic acids like vinegar may improve gut health in poultry, and vinegar won't hurt if you give it at the recommended dose. Any kind of vinegar will do, although you probably

> won't want to use your $50 bottle of artisan balsamic. Chickens don't seem to notice it at this recommended dose.
>
> ✔ **Use a probiotic medication or offer yogurt.** Most feed stores sell probiotics that you can add to feed or water. The organisms in yogurt and probiotics compete with the bad bugs, and sometimes the good bugs win.

Tetracycline medications (such as oxytetracycline, chlortetracycline) are commonly used in drinking water or feed to successfully treat diarrhea in livestock, including chickens. As a result of that common use, tetracycline medications just as frequently fail to cure diarrhea because bacteria are now often resistant to the drug. If you're a U.S. flock keeper, and you want to use an antibiotic for laying hens, you need to get a prescription and an egg discard time from a veterinarian if you want to stay on the right side of the law. An *egg discard time* is the number of days you need to throw out potentially contaminated eggs after you medicate a hen.

Egg-Laying Troubles: Egg-Binding and Vent Prolapse

A hen having trouble laying eggs is *egg-bound.* When part of a hen's *oviduct* (which should stay inside the abdomen; see Chapter 2) sticks out through the vent to the outside, the hen is suffering from a *vent prolapse, oviduct prolapse,* or more graphically, a *blowout.* We discuss vent prolapse and egg-binding conditions together in these sections, because this is a chicken-and-egg situation.

Identifying vent prolapse and egg-binding

A hen who spends a lot of time in the nest box is *broody,* not egg-bound. Broodiness is the compelling feeling a hen gets to sit and incubate eggs. An egg-bound hen, on the other hand, strains to pass an egg repeatedly throughout the day (in or out of the nest box), wagging or bobbing her tail with the effort.

You rarely discover which came first — whether difficulty laying an egg resulted in a vent prolapse or the other way around. Either way, the common causes of egg-binding and vent prolapses are

✔ Obesity

✔ Poor diet

✔ A tendency to lay very big or misshaped eggs (especially rubbery ones)

✔ Oviduct infections

✔ *Egg peritonitis* (a nasty, often fatal infection inside the abdomen)

See Chapter 11 for tips on slimming down spoiled hens, and Chapter 12 for a discussion of egg peritonitis, in the section on *colibacillosis.*

Providing treatment and care

You have the best chance of successfully treating these two conditions when you place the care of the bird in the hands of an experienced avian or exotic pet veterinarian, because he or she frequently treats these two problems in pet birds and reptiles. If egg-binding or vent prolapses are caught early, avian and exotic pet vets can medically treat these conditions, or if necessary, do surgery. Hysterectomy is the best option for a beloved pet hen who has repeated episodes of egg-binding. (It also ends her egg-laying career.)

If experienced professional help isn't an option, flock keepers may be able to help an egg-bound or prolapsed hen by following these steps:

1. **Isolate the affected bird in a quiet hospital pen by herself and provide TLC.**

   Maintain the temperature in the hospital pen at a consistent, comfortable 80–85 degrees Fahrenheit (27–29 degrees Celsius). Feed a complete commercial layer diet — no junk food or scratch. Offer oyster shell, available at feed stores, or crushed egg shells (available at home) as a calcium supplement. Provide a low, comfortable perch, and keep the bedding in the hospital pen super-clean. Frequently changing the bedding with clean towels may be the best option because most types of litter sticks to the hen's backside.

2. **Soak the chicken's lower half in warm water.**

   Make the bath water as warm as you would bathe in. Carefully cleanse a dirty vent in the water. Gently restrain the hen in the bath as long as she doesn't mind it or until the water cools. Ten to twenty minutes of soaking is a good goal. If she freaks out, put her back in the hospital pen and leave her alone for a while.

3. **Gently apply a water-based lubricant on the vent and protruding tissues.**

   Use a plain, nonscented, nonmedicated lubricant, available at any drugstore. You can make a brief, one-time attempt to gently push protruding tissues back in with clean fingers. More often than not, the darn thing will pop out again. After that attempt, succeed or fail, leave a prolapse alone. The more you handle her or rub the inflamed tissues with various ointments, the more swollen the area will become.

4. **Leave her alone.**

   Let her relax without other animals or people pestering her. Shrinkage of a prolapse or passage of a stuck egg within 24 hours is a good sign. No progress in 24 hours is grim news. Keep the hen isolated for several days until she seems perkier and the vent area looks normal.

Give the oviduct a break for a while by slowing egg production. You can do this by keeping the hen in the dark for 16 hours a day.

Popping Out Strange Eggs: Egg Quality Issues

A star-performer backyard hen can lay more than 250 eggs a year, but even superstars have occasional bad days, and not all of her eggs will be perfect. Some of the eggs from healthy hens are really weird: soft, rubbery, sandpapery, or lumpy, for example. Hens that consistently lay abnormal eggs, however, are likely to have a problem somewhere in the plumbing of the reproductive tract. (We describe the normal functioning of that plumbing in Chapter 2.) Here we discuss what causes these weird eggs and what you can do about them when you notice them.

Finding the cause

A multitude of factors can cause abnormal eggshell shape and texture. The amount of time the egg spends in the shell gland of the oviduct determines the thickness and shape of the shell. Anything — such as age, stress, nutrition, or viral infections — that speeds up or slows down the normal transit time through the shell gland will result in shell abnormalities. We provide possible causes of commonly seen strange eggs in Table 8-3.

Table 8-3	Egg Quality Problems and Causes	
Egg Defect	*Possible Causes*	*Possible Remedies*
Thin shell	Egg laid later in the day Hot weather Older hen Hen in lay for a year or more Poor diet, often a diet low in calcium	Get younger hens Allow older hens to molt by decreasing daily hours of light Provide complete layer diet and offer oyster shell
Soft or no shell	A scare or a stressful event Infectious bronchitis, Newcastle disease, or other infection of the oviduct Poor diet, often a diet low in calcium	Eliminate stress Handle hens gently Provide complete layer diet Vaccinate new pullets
Blood-stained shell	Young hen Underweight hen Vent picking	Provide complete layer diet Use feather-pecking prevention methods (See Chapter 11)
Sandpaper texture, lumps, or chalky coating on shell	Stress Young hen Hen delayed in laying an egg	Eliminate stress Provide more nest boxes
Body checks (ridges on shell) or a bulge around the "equator" of the egg	Egg cracked inside the oviduct	Provide more space for hens Handle hens gently
Brown egg layers suddenly lay white or blotchy eggs Shell crinkles Watery whites	Infectious bronchitis, Newcastle disease, or other infection of the oviduct	No treatment for affected hens Vaccinate new pullets

An abnormal egg every once in a while is — well — normal. Some egg oddities, like double-yolkers or no-yolkers, are just accidents (or maybe a hen's sense of humor?). Don't worry about it. On the other hand, if you suddenly get many strange eggs, or if several members of the flock lay them consistently, that calls for an investigation.

Handling odd-shaped eggs with care

If you identify odd-shaped eggs, don't be overly concerned unless it reoccurs with the same chicken for a long time or happens to several members of the flock at one time. Poultry scientists at agricultural colleges can provide a lot of information about egg quality problems. Veterinary diagnostic laboratories can run tests for viral infections in the flock.

Eggs with ugly shells are unappealing to you and your customers, but they're okay for people to eat after cooking. Eggs with defective shells are more prone to breaking and invisible cracks, which reduce the egg's shelf life. Incubate only perfect-looking eggs for the best success in hatching.

Seeing Trouble: Poor Sight and Sore Eyes

Chickens have extremely good daytime vision. In fact, chickens rely on their sense of sight more than other senses to conduct their daily business. Flock keepers notice quickly when chickens have impaired vision and aren't able to cope with finding food, navigating the coop, or avoiding bullies. That's when they take a closer look at the chicken's eyes, and find . . . What *is* that? You may find it difficult to describe an eye problem or identify the part of the eye that's affected, due to unfamiliarity with the anatomy. These sections give you a rundown on chicken eye anatomy, point out some causes of chicken eye problems, and suggest ways to deal with them.

Eyeing potential eye problems

In this section, we describe the parts of a chicken's eye in a little more detail and point out causes of eye problems of adult chickens, by location. Figure 8-2 shows parts of the eye to help you get your bearings. Refer to Chapter 2 for a discussion about the rest of a chicken's anatomy.

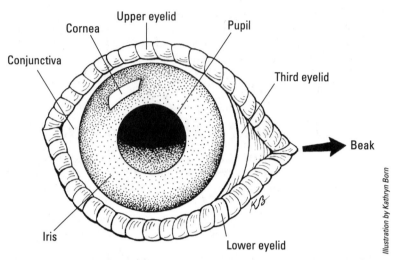

Figure 8-2: The different parts of a chicken's eye.

✔ **Eyelids:** A chicken's eye has three eyelids — upper, lower, and the third eyelid.

Fowl pox, a viral infection, causes scabby eyelids. See Chapter 12 for prevention and supportive care for cases of fowl pox.

✔ **Conjunctiva:** This is the moist, pink tissue around the eye. Inflammation of this tissue is known as *conjunctivitis,* or *pink eye.*

• Small stuff *(foreign bodies)* like seeds or grit can get stuck in the conjunctiva.

• Conjunctivitis usually goes along with respiratory infections, which we describe in the "Sneezing and Coughing: Chicken Head Colds" section earlier in this chapter.

• Eyeworms cause swollen conjunctiva in chickens living in the tropics and possibly in warmer areas of the United States. See Chapter 13 for more information about this parasite.

✔ **Cornea:** This is the transparent front part of the eye that covers the iris and the pupil. An injured cornea is very painful, so the chicken will hold the eye shut. A damaged cornea may become cloudy. If you find it difficult to see the iris or the pupil through a cloudy eye, the cornea is mostly likely the location of the problem.

A cloudy cornea may be the result of an injury or an infection with bacteria, a virus, or a fungus. Ammonia fumes from dirty, wet litter can injure the cornea. Cloudy corneas can get better, or turn into permanent scars.

✔ **Iris:** It's the colored part of the eye, which is commonly reddish brown in chickens. The irises of both eyes should be the same color. Here's a strange, but commonly seen iris defect:

An iris that turns gray (called *gray eye*) is a sign of Marek's disease (Chapter 12).

✔ **Pupil:** The *pupil* is the round dark spot in the center of the eye that lets light through to the back of the eye. The pupil should be round, have distinct (not blurry) edges, and get smaller if you shine a light on the eye. The following are not-quite-right chicken pupils:

- An irregularly shaped (not round) pupil is a sign of Marek's disease (Chapter 12).

- A white spot or cloudy look to the pupil may be a *cataract,* which is often the result of avian encephalomyelitis infection as a chick (Chapter 12), vitamin A deficiency (Chapter 11), old age, or genetics.

Getting treatment for eye issues

A veterinary ophthalmologist, a specialist who does nothing but look at animal eyes all day, is the go-to person for state-of-the-art care of a troublesome eye problem in a pet chicken. You won't find an eye vet in most towns, but any small animal veterinarian will be able to refer you to the closest veterinary ophthalmologist.

We suggest you try these simple treatment options if you identify minor issues:

✔ **Conjunctiva:** If your hen has something in her eye, you can flush out the gunky eye with an eye wash, which may help dislodge a foreign body. A dilute boric acid solution is an old remedy for pink eye; see the appendix for a recipe.

✔ **Cornea:** In the early stages of a cornea injury, applying an antibiotic ointment to the affected eye twice daily may be helpful. A do-it-yourselfer can purchase tetracycline ophthalmic ointment at pet or farm supply stores or online.

✔ **Iris:** No treatment is available for Marek's disease and gray eye.

✔ **Pupil:** Irregular pupils and cataracts also don't have any treatment.

Poor vision due to swelling of the eyelid, conjunctiva, or cornea can get better as the swelling subsides. Blindness due to Marek's disease, cataracts, or scarred corneas is permanent. A chicken blind in one eye often does well with the handicap. It's your judgment call whether a blind chicken is coping; you can use the body condition scoring system in Chapter 7 to keep tabs on the bird's ability to eat and fit in with the rest of the flock.

Digging into Skin Problems and Feather Loss

Molting is a normal, orderly process of feather loss that chickens go through annually, usually in the fall (See Chapter 2 for more information about molt). Your molting chicken needs no special help from you other than your normal care and attention.

On the other hand, overbearing flock mates or skin diseases can be making your chicken's feathers fall out. These sections will help you tell the difference between normal and abnormal feather loss, and help you deal with true skin problems.

Noticing feather and skin issues

Molt is no cause for alarm, but other reasons for feather loss may be serious problems, so you need to distinguish between normal and abnormal feather loss. Here's how to tell the difference: Feather loss during molt moves in a wave over the chicken's body, roughly in a head-to-tail direction, and the chicken has a bright new suit of feathers in little more than a month. Lots of short, stiff, tube-shaped pinfeathers emerge where feathers have been shed.

Molt doesn't cause scabby, bumpy, lumpy, or sore skin. Tiny, unidentified scurrying objects on the skin aren't a normal part of molt. Droopiness, swollen eyes, or loss of appetite aren't expected, either; birds feel fine when they are molting. We provide non-molt common causes of feather loss and skin problems in Table 8-4.

Table 8-4 Feather Loss and Skin Problems in Adult Chickens

Problem	Location	Possible Causes
Feather loss	Head, neck, or shoulders	Feather pecking by flock mates Poking head through fence wire
	Hen's breast	Normal in a broody hen
	Hen's back	Attention from rooster
	Vent area	Feather pecking by flock mates
	Patchy all over	Louse infestation
Scabby skin	Non-feathered areas (comb, wattles, face, eyelids)	Fowl pox
	Feathered areas	Tumors caused by Marek's disease
	Vent or tail area	Mite infestation
White bumps or nodules on skin	Feathered areas	Tumors caused by Marek's disease
White clumps at base of feathers' shafts	Anywhere on body	Louse infestation
Dirty-looking patches of clumped feathers	Anywhere on body	Mite infestation

Soothing skin problems

We suggest remedies for feather pecking in Chapter 11 and for mites and lice in Chapter 13. Giving some TLC can help birds recover from fowl pox, a viral disease that we describe in Chapter 12. You can also give your hens with bald backs a break by moving the rooster out for a while, or you can try cloth saddles to protect the hens' backs. Tumors caused by Marek's disease are incurable, and the outcome of Marek's disease in unvaccinated chickens is usually fatal.

Focusing on a Dizzy Chicken and Other Alarming Signs

Chickens aren't known for their smarts; "bird-brain" isn't a complimentary term, after all. Still, that tiny lump of gray matter between a chicken's ears and the network of nerves throughout the rest of the body are critical pieces of anatomy, if not for advanced problem solving, then definitely for good balance and nimble beak and claw action.

If a chicken's brain or nerves go haywire, for any number of reasons, the chicken can experience alarming signs of paralysis, lack of coordination, and other nervous system disorders. A chicken that can't move about, scratch, and peck with dexterity can't make a living, so brain and nerve problems are serious issues. You can prevent some of these disorders and treat just a few of them, which is why we share that information with you in the following sections.

Mapping out nervous system issues

You may see the following signs when infection, inflammation, injury, toxicity, or tumors affect the nervous system (brain and nerves) of a chicken:

- Dizziness, staggering, or incoordination
- *Torticollis* (the neck is held in a twisted, abnormal position)
- Paralysis of one or both legs or wings (the bird is unable to walk or has a droopy wing)
- Weakness, whole body paralysis, or coma
- Twitching or flopping
- Blindness

Unfortunately, these frightening signs of illness aren't unusual in backyard flocks. Each of the diseases in Table 8-5 can cause one or more nervous systems signs in adult chickens. In the table, we also list some distinctive signs for each disease that may help you determine the most likely diagnosis. The number of affected birds in the flock gives you a clue to the cause; for example, ingested toxins usually affect many birds in the flock in a short period of time, because chickens don't like to dine alone.

Table 8-5	Some Nervous System Diseases of Adult Chickens		
Disease	*Occurrence*	*Distinctive Signs*	*Typical Number of Birds Affected in a Flock*
Marek's disease	Common	Torticollis, limping on one leg, paralysis of any part, split leg posture	Few
Botulism	Common	Progresses to whole body paralysis, including eyelids	Many
Abdominal tumor or egg peritonitis	Common	Paralysis or limping on one leg in an older hen	One
Bacterial infection in the brain	Not so common	Torticollis, coma, blindness	One
Toxicity from pesticides or drugs	Not so common	Twitching, staggering, coma	Many
Bacterial infection in the spine	Not so common	Paralysis of both legs *(dog-sitting posture)*	One
Toxic plants	Rare	Varies	Few
Some strains of Newcastle disease and avian influenza	Rare (not present in the United States)	Weakness, staggering, torticollis, diarrhea, and respiratory signs	Many

Marek's disease, which can cause nearly any combination of the nervous system signs we list, is probably the most common cause of brain and nerve disease in backyard flocks. For more details about the menace of Marek's and other viral threats, such as Newcastle disease and avian influenza, see Chapter 12. We discuss botulism and other nervous system diseases caused by toxins in Chapter 11.

A veterinary diagnostic laboratory will be the most helpful resource for you to diagnose a nervous system illness in a bird or a flock. Check out Chapter 15 for tips on submitting dead or sick birds to a laboratory.

Reacting to nervous system problems

If you suspect that a toxin is affecting your flock and causing your flock's nervous system issues, do the following in order:

- ✔ Immediately eliminate any suspected source.

- ✔ You can then use an Epsom salt laxative to help the birds eliminate the toxin faster. See the appendix for a laxative solution and dosing to treat individual chickens or the whole flock in the drinking water.

- ✔ Isolate sick birds away from the rest of the flock. We describe a hospital cage set-up and good nursing care for sick birds in Chapter 17.

Limping or Swelling: Leg and Foot Issues

You may not have been watching when your hen sprinted away from a swooping hawk, or escaped from the rooster's amorous advances. Maybe your suddenly limping hen just strained something, but maybe a more sinister issue is afoot. In these sections, we help you pin down the location of a leg or foot problem, so that you can close in on a diagnosis and quickly address the problem.

Zooming in on your chicken's leg and foot pains

Check over your limping chicken using the following pointers:

- ✔ If she's bearing some weight on the leg, a broken bone or ruptured tendon is unlikely. A chicken is usually unable to use a broken leg at all, and the bird may use a wing for some support and balance.

- ✔ Look at the bottom of her foot. Do you see a sore or swollen foot pad? If so, your bird has *bumblefoot,* which is a bacterial infection in the footpad that may be the result of a puncture wound, rough perches, or a wet, dirty pen. Read more about bumblefoot in Chapter 14.

✔ Stroke the feathers of the leg backward, or blow on the feathers to reveal the skin of the leg and thigh. Do you see any puncture wounds, cuts, or bruising? We provide some DIY advice for treating injuries in Chapter 17.

✔ If you can get someone else to help you hold the bird up facing you, pull gently on both feet to extend the legs and compare them side by side. They should be symmetrical. Do you see any difference between the injured and uninjured leg, such as a bigger hock joint or swollen toe? A swollen joint may be the result of a viral or bacterial infection, and the damage done by the infectious organism may or may not be permanent. A leg that appears bent, compared to the other leg, may have suffered a tendon injury or broken bone.

Limping in an adult bird is often an early sign of Marek's disease, which is incurable. If so, you probably won't see anything out of the ordinary when you examine the leg. After a few days of limping for no apparent reason, a bird with Marek's disease may appear to recover, only to die of tumors a short time later. See Chapter 12 for information about preventing Marek's disease in your flock.

Seeking treatment help

Avian veterinarians are the pros to turn to for help with bumblefoot, joint infections, broken bones, and tendon injuries. If you suspect something minor (the chased-by-hawk scenario, maybe) and want to try supportive care at home for a few days, we suggest the following steps:

1. **Isolate the bird in a small area, so she doesn't need to move much, and won't get picked on.**

   Don't provide a perch until she's improved. See our nursing care suggestions in Chapter 17.

2. **Give aspirin in the drinking water for two to three days**.

   See the appendix for dose and mixing instructions.

Using antibiotics for chicken joint infections is tricky these days, because antibiotic resistance is so common among bacteria such as *Staphylococcus* or *Streptococcus* that usually cause these infections. A veterinarian working with a diagnostic laboratory can identify the bacteria infecting a joint and determine which antibiotic is likely to work, but this testing may not be feasible for most flock keepers. You can try erythromycin, lincomycin, or tetracycline, but you need to get a prescription and an egg discard time from a veterinarian in order to treat laying hens.

Chapter 9

Sizing Up Sick Chicks

After you bring home a few adorable, fluffy chicks for the first time, you'll soon be bitten by the poultry-raising bug. Before you know it, you'll want to hatch your own chicks and buy your own incubator and brooder. When the first incubator fills up, you'll have to buy another, and then. . . . We understand, because we also share the obsession and delight of hatching and raising chicks.

Chicks are sturdy, precocious infants by animal kingdom standards, and they're typically easy to raise and forgiving of minor mistakes of novice caretakers. Things can go wrong, however, and eventually, if you hatch enough chicks (who can resist?), you'll encounter a problem with a hatchling or a growing bird. We hope this chapter can help when that happens. We cover the major pediatric problems that backyard flock keepers see, from hatch day to the time a pullet thinks about laying her first egg, around 4 months of age.

Before Hatching: Ensuring a Healthy Chick

Success in incubation is mostly a matter of obtaining clean, fertile eggs from a healthy, well-fed flock and incubating them at the proper temperature and humidity in a clean incubator. Easier said than done, right? Your incubator's instruction manual is the best reference for temperature and humidity specifications for your particular model.

Cleanliness of the hatching eggs and the incubator, along with proper temperature, humidity, and ventilation are the important factors that you can control. See Chapter 5 for tips on cleaning and disinfection of poultry equipment, including incubators and hatching trays.

Set only perfect, unwashed eggs for hatching in your incubator. A perfect, unwashed hatching egg is a beauty of symmetry and size (not too big and not too small), with no cracks or other imperfections, and so clean you wouldn't mind licking it. If you keep the parent flock, you can make sure the eggs are super-clean right out of the nest with the tips in Chapter 20.

If you purchase hatching eggs, you don't have control over the nutrition or health of the breeder flock, but you can select pullorum-free parents for your chicks. *Pullorum* is a serious egg-transmitted disease, now rare in the United States, which kills many hatchlings; see Chapter 12 for more information. Ask the flock keeper if the parent flock is certified free of pullorum disease. In the United States, that certification is part of the National Poultry Improvement Plan (NPIP).

We highly recommend that you dabble in the art of *candling,* shining a light through an egg to view its contents, as a way to evaluate fertility and embryo development during incubation. Many online resources show you how to candle eggs. A bright LED flashlight is a fantastic (and inexpensive) improvement over old-school incandescent candling lamps.

Spotting Problems of the Newly Hatched

The starting point in a chick's life is *pipping,* the moment that a chick breaks through the shell and begins its entrance into the world. You can sit back and watch with amazement as the chick wins its freedom from the shell with a determined series of in-egg gymnastic movements. A healthy hatchling innately knows exactly what to do, and you shouldn't interfere with the program. The moment for you to step in is immediately after hatching, when you have a role in preventing four common problems of the newly hatched, which are chick malformations, spraddle legs, belly button infections, and pasty vents. We tell you how to give your hatchlings the best shot at growing up healthy.

Finding reasons for chick malformations

After waiting with excitement for your chicks to hatch, your heart sinks when you see a malformed chick emerge. What could have gone wrong? You may not have been able to prevent it. Even under ideal conditions, approximately one out of 250 chicks hatched will have a deformity. Table 9-1 lists common malformations and some known causes for them, which fall into categories of genetic traits, incubation errors, and nutritional deficiencies. You may not be able to help an abnormal chick after it's hatched, but you can correct incubator settings and possibly flock nutrition to avoid some deformities next time you set eggs to hatch (refer to the previous section).

Table 9-1	Common Chick Malformations and Causes
Malformation	*Possible Causes*
Beak abnormalities, such as crossed beak, parrot beak, or short upper beak	Genetic trait
	Poor hen nutrition
	Exposure to pesticide
	Hatching eggs exposed to near freezing temperatures
Small or missing eye(s)	High temperature during incubation
Exposed brain	High temperature during early incubation
Intestines outside of abdomen	High temperature during mid-incubation
	Hatching eggs exposed to near freezing temperatures
Crooked (wry) neck	Genetic trait Poor hen nutrition
Crooked toes	Poor hen nutrition Genetic trait

Chick malformations with nutritional causes were much more common back when complete commercial diets weren't available and flock keepers had to prepare their own homemade chicken feed. Breeder hens fed a complete commercial layer diet rarely produce chicks with malformations related to nutritional deficiencies, such as lack of B vitamins or zinc. Finding many malformations in batches of hatchlings calls for an investigation into the vitamin and mineral content of the parent flock's diet.

Most malformed chicks have a poor chance of becoming healthy, productive members of a backyard flock. Many, but not all chick malformations can be inherited traits, so malformed chicks who survive should not be used for breeding because they can pass on the trait to future generations. For these reasons, euthanizing a malformed chick is justifiable, if done humanely. We give advice about euthanasia of chicks in Chapter 18.

Straightening spraddled legs

Although most chick malformations aren't correctable, one very common abnormality of newly hatched chicks called *spraddle leg* responds very well to treatment. You can create the problem of spraddle leg by allowing chicks to hatch on surfaces that are too smooth — newspaper or cardboard are the common culprits.

A chick can't get traction to stand and walk on a slick floor, and as a result, the legs splay outward as in Figure 9-1. Other than the odd pose, the chick looks alert and acts normally; however, the chick won't get better and be able to walk without your help. Here's how you do it:

1. **Place the chick on a surface with more texture so that the chick can get a grip with its feet**.

   Straw, shavings, and wire mesh are good choices.

2. **Bring the legs back together in a normal position using a bandage between the legs.**

   A three-quarter inch adhesive bandage is perfect for the job. Cut the bandage lengthwise down the middle. Place the pad of the bandage between the legs, and then wrap the sticky ends of the bandage around each leg just above the foot; see Figure 9-1. Cloth bandage tape, masking tape, or a piece of yarn work as well.

3. **Leave the bandage on for two days.**

   Usually, you can leave the bandaged chick in the brooder with the hatch mates during this time. The other chicks will encourage the bandaged chick to move around and get stronger.

4. **After two days, remove the bandage and see if the chick can walk normally.**

   If not, reapply a bandage for two more days. A chick that isn't walking normally at four days of age is unlikely to improve, so unfortunately, you should euthanize that chick to prevent the suffering that lies ahead.

Singing the belly-button blues

If your incubator is set in the Goldilocks zone — not too warm, not too hot, humidity and ventilation just right — your chicks will either hatch with properly healed navels, or the navels will finish closing up in the first hour or so after hatching, as the chick dries off and fluffs up. Poorly healed navels are a sign that conditions in the incubator weren't ideal. Table 9-2 shows belly-button problems and the incubator errors that can cause them.

Table 9-2   Chick Belly-Button Problems and Causes

Problem	*Possible Causes*
Poorly closed navels	High humidity during incubation
	Low temperature during the last few days of incubation
Navels with a string of dried tissue attached	Low temperature during incubation
Bloody navels or navels that look like black buttons	High temperature during incubation
Blood on eggshells or hatcher trays	High temperature during incubation

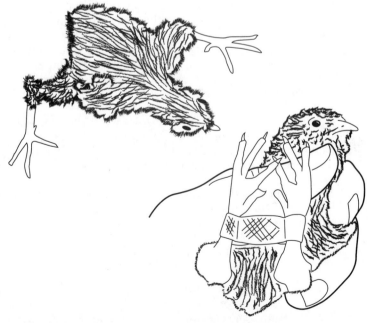

Illustration by Barbara Frake

Figure 9-1: A chick with spraddle leg and a bandage to correct the condition.

An unhealed navel leaves the door open for bacteria from the environment to invade and infect a chick. If you hatched a batch of chicks that had many unhealed navels, be obsessive about cleanliness in the brooder in order to prevent infections.

Probably the most common cause of chick death in the first week of hatching is *omphalitis,* an infection of the navel and yolk sac, also known as navel ill or mushy chick disease. Omphalitis is the reason to be concerned about unhealed navels, which predispose chicks to the infection. Chicks begin to die from omphalitis the first day after hatching, and deaths may continue until the chicks are about 8 days old. You may not see any signs of illness prior to death, but if you do, you'll see a drowsy, droopy chick who has no appetite. The chick's abdomen may look swollen or feel mushy, and you may see bluish discoloration in the navel area or discharge with a bad odor.

Unfortunately, chicks in this state are almost always past any help; even a broad-spectrum antibiotic, such as gentamicin, which some flock keepers use to prevent omphalitis, isn't likely to save them at this late stage in the illness. All you can do is focus on prevention for the next batch. Make sure you set only clean eggs in the incubator and pay close attention to temperature, humidity, and ventilation settings.

Unpasting a pasty vent

Just like grown-up birds, chicks with diarrhea have messy vents (refer to Chapter 8 for more information). Watery droppings accumulate around the vent, and the caked-up poop may even plug the opening. You may even see the back end of the chick bulge with the pressure of the backed-up poop. Pasty vent is rare in chicks raised by momma hen, but it's a common condition in artificially incubated and brooded chicks. With some TLC from you, most chicks with pasty vent can survive.

A pasty vent isn't a stand-alone disease; it's a sign, telling you something is wrong in the brooder where you keep your baby chicks. Chilling or overheating is the most common cause of pasty vent, but viral or bacterial infections or poor diet can trigger it, too.

After adjusting the temperature in the brooder area to 90–95 degrees Fahrenheit (32–35 degrees Celsius), here are the steps for dealing with a chick with a pasty vent:

1. **Soak the pasted-up behind in warm, clean water for a minute or two to soften the gunk**.

   Do this in a warm, nondrafty place to avoid chilling the chick. Use clean water as warm as you would bathe in. Don't soak the whole chick — just the butt.

2. **Gently peel away the caked droppings**.

   It's okay if a few down feathers come with the lump. If the dried poop is still very hard to remove, soak again.

3. **Apply a little vegetable oil or mineral oil to the vent area.**

   Don't use diaper rash cream containing zinc or other remedies you wouldn't want the other chicks to eat, because they will pick at it! Promptly put the chick back in the brooder to warm up. Keep an eye on the chick because you may need to separate the chick from the others if they pick at the vent area.

4. **Keep chlorinated water in the chick waterer.**

   Doing so may limit spread of an infection in the group of chicks through the water. Check the appendix for instructions on mixing the solution. Antibiotics aren't helpful or recommended for pasty vent. Offering yogurt or another probiotic isn't a bad idea.

Recognizing Problems of Growing Chickens

You make it through your chicks' first week of life. So are you out of the woods? Not yet. More perils of chickhood lurk around the corner, but many are fortunately preventable and some are treatable. The most common problems of the growing period of backyard chickens' lives are

- ✔ Respiratory illness
- ✔ Diarrhea
- ✔ Nervous system signs

We discuss these three in greater depth in the following sections. Young chickens can suffer from all the causes of respiratory illness in adult birds that we list in Chapter 8. Diagnosis and treatment are also the same as we describe for adult birds.

Suffering from respiratory problems

Brooder pneumonia and gapeworms are two special respiratory problems of chicks that aren't usually seen in grown-up chickens in backyard flocks. Symptoms include the following:

✔ **Brooder pneumonia:** Gasping, rapid breathing, and drowsiness are typical signs of this condition in chicks; see Chapter 14 for more detail about brooder pneumonia.

✔ **Gapeworms:** When a chick has gapeworms, the infested young bird gasps for air with outstretched necks; we discuss gapeworm infections in Chapter 13.

Dealing with diarrhea in young chickens

Coccidiosis is guilty, until proven innocent, in cases of diarrhea in young chickens. The intestinal disease, caused by parasites called *coccidia,* is enemy number one for poultry raisers around the world. We describe coccidiosis in detail in Chapter 13, and we list treatments for it in the appendix.

If you see runny poop or blood in the droppings of young chickens, promptly begin treatment for coccidiosis. In backyard flocks, young chickens sick with coccidiosis get better quickly with anticoccidial medication. Without treatment, many affected birds will die.

You rarely need to look any further than the first row in Table 9-3 for the cause of diarrhea in young chickens, but we include a few other fairly common causes just to be thorough. Veterinarians and veterinary diagnostic laboratories can perform examinations of droppings for parasites and perform postmortems to help you get a diagnosis for your birds' intestinal trouble.

Table 9-3 Common Causes of Diarrhea in Young Chickens

Disease	Age Typically Affected	Distinctive Signs of Illness
Coccidiosis (see Chapter 13)	3–5 weeks	Bloody droppings, more common in warm weather
Roundworms and threadworms (see Chapter 13)	1–3 months	Not gaining weight despite a good appetite
Necrotic enteritis (see Chapter 12)	2–5 weeks	Depression, sudden death, more common in warm weather
Infectious bursal disease (see Chapter 12)	3–6 weeks	Watery diarrhea, inflamed vents, staggering

Identifying nervous system illnesses in young chickens

A dizzy chicken sounds like a comical concept for a video shared online, but we have nothing funny to say about the miserable diseases affecting the brain and nerves of young chickens. Young chickens with nervous system disorders can show the same signs that we describe for adult birds in Chapter 8: staggering, incoordination, weakness, paralysis of one or both legs and wings, or twisted neck. If the disease progresses, eventually a chick with a damaged nervous system may not be able to get up to eat and drink, and its flock mates may trample it.

Birds of any age can show nervous system signs due to viral or bacterial infections, or botulism and other toxins (see Chapter 11 for more discussion). Marek's disease and avian encephalomyelitis are two diseases that unfortunately are often found in young chickens in backyard flocks. Two nutritional disorders, vitamin B1 (thiamine) deficiency and crazy chick disease caused by vitamin E deficiency, occasionally pop up, usually in flocks fed poorly balanced homemade diets. We compare nervous system diseases of young chickens in Table 9-4.

Table 9-4   Nervous System Disorders of Young Chickens

Disease	Age Typically Affected	Distinctive Signs of Illness	Mortality Rate in Affected Birds
Marek's disease	Older than 6 weeks	Lameness, twisted neck, droopy wing, paralysis with one leg forward and one leg back, or wasting	Nearly 100 percent
Avian encephalomyelitis (AE)	2–16 weeks	Trembling of the head, paralysis with both legs held out to one side	25–60 percent
Crazy chick disease (vitamin E deficiency)	2–4 weeks	Chick is unable to walk, falls on its side, or stands with head between its legs; head may also twist sideways or over the back	Depends on severity of deficiency
Vitamin B1 deficiency	Less than 1 week	Chick can't stand and draws its head back into a star-gazing position	Depends on severity of deficiency

The best chance of making an exact diagnosis is ultimately through postmortem examination and testing of dead birds at a veterinary diagnostic laboratory.

No treatment for Marek's disease or avian encephalomyelitis exists for affected birds, although vaccinating and raising young birds in isolation may prevent the illnesses. You can treat crazy chick disease with a vitamin E supplement; some chicks will get better, but some will be left with a permanent head tilt or other nervous system disorder. Vitamin B1 deficiency is the most treatable of the four diseases; chicks given vitamin B1 by mouth usually bounce back within hours. Read more about these two nutritional disorders in Chapter 11, and the two viral illnesses, Marek's disease and avian encephalomyelitis, in Chapter 12.

We recommend two steps for treatment of an affected young chicken at home, if a trip to a veterinarian isn't an option:

1. **Isolate the young chicken and provide good nursing care.**

   We describe TLC for chickens in Chapter 17.

2. **Administer a vitamin supplement.**

   Give 1 mL (about a quarter teaspoon) of a liquid vitamin supplement by mouth drop by drop. The vitamin solution should contain vitamins A, B complex, D3, and E — other vitamins or iron won't hurt as a single dose.

   You can find a vitamin supplement formulated for poultry at a feed store, or in a pinch, you can use a child's liquid multivitamin. After the emergency dose, use a vitamin-electrolyte solution for poultry in the drinking water and feed a chick starter or grower diet.

Chapter 10

Sleuthing Subtle Signs of Illness and Mysterious Sudden Death

. . . .

In This Chapter

▶ Knowing when your chicken is sick (and when it isn't)

▶ Puzzling over the flock owner's nightmare: sudden death in chickens

. . . .

Subtle and sudden are the chicken illnesses we tackle in this chapter. First, we discuss the ADR chicken with a vague, lingering problem, such as stunted growth, weight loss, or decreased egg production. What's ADR? ADR is highly technical jargon that veterinarians write in the medical record of an animal with subtle signs of illness that defy diagnosis — ADR stands for "Ain't doin' right." At the other abrupt end of the chicken illness spectrum (and the chapter) is sudden death. We provide you with a list of suspects and encourage you to conduct some veterinary detective work to close the case.

Veterinarians have a saying, "When you hear hoof beats, think horses, not zebras." The problem you're seeing or hearing (the sound of a stampede approaching) nearly always has a common cause, so you should rule out the usual suspects (horses) before expecting a herd of zebras to gallop onto the scene. To help you in your search for a cause of an obscure chicken health problem, we list possibilities as common, not-so-common, or rare in chickens living in North American backyards.

We can't list all the possibilities for vague illnesses and sudden death in chickens, just the ones that are better understood, or that we've witnessed personally. People understand quite a bit about some chicken health problems, but unfortunately other illnesses are mysteries that veterinarians don't know a lot about. In addition, chickens don't read books, so they may show unexpected or atypical signs and fool everyone. For these reasons, you may find it difficult, maybe impossible, to discover an exact cause for your chicken's illness. Your best chance in finding the cause for the problems in this chapter is through some detective work and with the help of a veterinary diagnostic laboratory or a veterinarian who works with poultry.

Investigating Not-So-Obvious Signs of Illness

If you're scratching your head, wondering what's not quite right about a chicken in your flock, read on. We may have some ideas. The most common, hard-to-put-your-finger-on-it problems in backyard flocks are poor growth in chicks, skinny adult chickens, and decreased egg production, which we discuss here.

Stunted growth in young chickens

Stunted young birds are small for their age and poorly feathered. The few feathers they do possess look ratty or stick out at crazy angles. A pale comb and drowsiness are clues that a stunted chick is anemic. A mind-boggling number of reasons can cause poor growth in chicks, and we list just a few in Table 10-1.

Table 10-1	Some Causes of Stunted Chicks		
Type of Disease	*Common Causes*	*Not-So-Common Causes*	*Rare Causes*
Accidents of flock management	High ammonia levels Water restriction	Nutritional deficiency, especially protein, vitamin A, salt	Low-level carbon monoxide poisoning
Bacteria or viruses (see Chapter 12)	Colibacillosis Mycoplasmosis	Chicken infectious anemia (CIA)	Pullorum disease Fowl typhoid
Parasites (see Chapter 13)	Coccidiosis Poultry mites or lice	Heavy infections with roundworms	Toxoplasmosis
Miscellaneous or mystery diseases (see Chapter 14)	Crop or gizzard impaction	Candidiasis	Infectious stunting syndrome

To troubleshoot the problem of one or more stunted chicks in a group of hatchlings, focus on the fixable first.

- ✔ **Make sure water is always available for chicks.** They won't eat well if they don't have water to drink.

- ✔ **Feed chicks a diet appropriate to growing birds' nutritional needs, especially in the amino acid and vitamin departments.** To take the guesswork out of chick nutrition, use a complete commercial *starter* diet. Refer to Chapter 6 for details about a starter diet.

- ✔ **Ensure the brooder area isn't closed up tight.** Good ventilation and clean bedding are very important to prevent buildup of ammonia gas and infections caused by poor sanitation.

- ✔ **Treat for common intestinal parasites of chicks.** The most common parasites are coccidia and roundworms. Even if coccidiosis isn't the primary cause of stunting (it often is), parasites are likely to attack chicks with weakened immune systems. You can treat coccidiosis with amprolium or sulfa-methazine medications in drinking water. Roundworms are also extremely common in chicks under three months old, and are easily treated. See Chapter 13 and the appendix for details and treatments.

An avian veterinarian is well-equipped to investigate causes of poor growth in a young chicken. If stunting is a flock-wide problem, you should enlist the help of a veterinary diagnostic laboratory. Euthanizing a chick or chicks who are doing poorly and having them examined may provide you with an answer that can save the rest of the flock.

Skinny hen or rooster

This type of chicken is skinny, maybe wasting away, which is about the only sign of a problem, as far as you can tell. Table 10-2 shows some possible causes for a skinny chicken with no other signs of illness.

Table 10-2	Causes of a Skinny Adult Chicken		
Type of Disease	*Common Causes*	*Not-So-Common Causes*	*Rare Causes*
Accidents of flock management (see Chapter 11)	Persecution by flock mates	Hardware disease or gizzard impaction Lead poisoning Vitamin A deficiency	Pasture plant toxicities
Bacteria or viruses (see Chapter 12)	Marek's disease Lymphoid leukosis	Avian tuberculosis	Fowl typhoid
Parasites (see Chapter 13)	Poultry mites and lice	Heavy infections with threadworms or tapeworms Coccidiosis	Toxoplasmosis

Because just about any disease that goes on for several weeks to several months can wear a chicken down and make the bird thin, do a thorough physical examination (see Chapter 7) to find other clues to the illness.

Table 10-2 is definitely a complicated list. If you have s sickly hen or rooster, where do you go from here? We suggest you start with the simplest, most treatable explanation first: A skinny hen may be on the bottom of the pecking order, and her bossy flock mates aren't allowing her to get her fair share of food. You can investigate and correct that situation (by making sure she gets her ample share of food and water) before you move down the list of possible diagnoses.

We suggest you follow this plan of action if you have a sickly hen (or rooster):

 1. **Separate the skinny hen and give her TLC in a hospital pen.**

    See Chapter 17 for tips on TLC. If the patient has a non-bossy hen friend, put her in the pen with her for company, because chickens fret when alone.

2. **Check the patient (and her friend) for mites or signs of other external parasites.**

   If you see signs of mites or lice, you need to treat the whole flock. See Chapter 13 for information about identifying and treating external parasites.

3. **Scout your flock's environment for things that shouldn't be there.**

   Chips of lead paint, short pieces of string, weeds, spoiled food, or loose bits of metal don't belong. Remove them before another chicken gets hurt.

After two weeks of your close attention, you should notice that the hen who just needed some "alone time" is gaining weight and doing better. If that's the case, you can try to reintroduce her to the flock. Before you put her back, though, add another feeder and provide the hen-pecked hen a sanctuary, such as a crate, box, or bushy area of the yard — someplace where she can escape the harassment if necessary.

What if she still looks rough, or even worse? For a pet chicken, consider a visit to an avian veterinarian. After a thorough examination, an avian veterinarian will want to perform blood tests, examine droppings, and take X-rays. On the other hand, if the main purpose of the flock is to produce eggs or meat, *culling* (euthanizing) a sickly hen and submitting the carcass to a veterinary diagnostic laboratory for examination is the best path to a diagnosis.

Armed with an accurate diagnosis from a veterinarian or a diagnostic laboratory, you may be able to take steps to prevent a problem that can affect the rest of your flock.

Decreasing egg production

You may wonder why your hens have stopped laying eggs, particularly in the autumn. Three completely routine reasons explain why a healthy hen lays fewer eggs, or stops laying altogether: molt, age, and decreasing daylight. The following bullets explain in greater detail:

- **About once a year, a hen molts her feathers and goes on vacation from laying eggs for several weeks.** *Molting* is a bird's regular and orderly process of shedding feathers to make way for new ones. A good layer usually lays eggs for 50 to 60 weeks, and then molts and takes a rest before returning to egg production. Poor layers and older hens molt more often and take longer to get back to business laying eggs.

Getting in touch with your daylight hours

Are your curious about the number of hours of daylight where you live so you can predict when short daylight hours (less than 14 hours) will slow your hens' egg production?

Check out this website: `http://aa.usno.navy.mil/data/docs/Dur_OneYear.php`. Enter your location and a daylight table will be calculated for you.

If you decide to use supplemental light in your coop, you can use the website to tell you what day in late summer you should start using artificial light, and when you'll be able to rely on all-natural light in the spring. Find the day on the chart when the hours of daylight drop below 14 hours — that's when you should start turning the lights on to keep up your hens' egg production through the cold months of the year.

✔ **A hen can live and lay eggs for many years, but her egg production declines as she ages.** A sharp drop in egg production occurs after she reaches three years of age. We've met a few 10-year-old hens who still lay an egg every once in a while. (In 2011, a 22-year-old hen living in Maryland held the record as the world's oldest living chicken.)

✔ **Hens need about 14 hours of daylight in order to maintain good egg production.** Hens exposed only to natural light stop laying eggs in the winter and return to producing eggs in the spring. If you want your hens to continue to lay eggs in the autumn and winter, you need to provide supplemental light in the coop.

A single 9-watt warm wavelength fluorescent bulb provides plenty of egg-laying stimulation for 200 square feet of coop floor space. Ideally, you should put coop lights on a timer so that the hens receive extra hours of light in the morning before sunrise. That way, the hens go to roost naturally with the sunset. (If you don't have electrical service in or near your coop, you can install a solar-powered shed light.)

 So if your hens aren't molting, it's high summer, and your egg production is down, what can you do? We suggest you do the following to examine the situation:

1. **Scout around and make sure the hens aren't fooling you by hiding eggs.**

   Look in unconventional nests, such as a forgotten corner of a shed or garage, or under intriguing and shady new landscaping plants. You may need to put the flock under

surveillance; predators may be stealing eggs, or hens may
have developed the terrible habit of egg-eating.

2. **Look at Table 10-3 for possible health problems that may
   be causing the drop in egg production.**

Table 10-3   Causes of Decreased Egg Production

Type of Disease	Common Causes	Not-So-Common Causes	Rare Causes
Accidents of flock management (see Chapter 11)	Heat stress Running out of feed Running out of water	Moldy feed Poor nutrition	Medication or pesticide toxicity Plant toxins
Bacteria or viruses (see Chapter 12)	Fowl pox Infectious bronchitis Infectious coryza Mycoplasmosis Newcastle disease	Avian encephalomyelitis	Avian influenza Fowl cholera
Parasites (see Chapter 13)	Poultry mites and lice	Coccidiosis Heavy infestations with roundworms, threadworms, or tapeworms	Fleas

3. **Make sure the hens always have fresh feed and water
   available and that they're comfortable.**

Hens need to be relaxed in order to produce lots of eggs.
Having enough fresh water and fresh feed is especially
important. Keep them comfortable in hot weather; we give
some cooling-off tips in Chapter 5. Furthermore, stress of
any kind can put hens off their game, so avoid moving them
around, or upsetting the social order by adding or removing birds. Ask your friend to leave the rambunctious dog at
home next time.

4. **Thoroughly examine as many birds as practical to find other clues.**

   We describe how to perform a physical examination in Chapter 7. You can spot mites and lice, which literally suck the life out of hard-working hens. Sneezing, coughing, and goopy eyes and nostrils usually go along with respiratory illnesses, such as mycoplasmosis and infectious coryza, which have a nasty side effect of decreasing egg production. Fowl pox produces scabby faces, combs, and wattles, along with a hit on egg production.

   A veterinary diagnostic laboratory or a veterinarian who works with poultry can perform blood tests to check for viral illnesses and examine droppings to identify low-grade parasite problems.

What Happened?! Investigating Sudden Death

Coming home to find one or more dead chickens in the pen is a flock keeper's nightmare. In this case, you're certain predators couldn't have done it; those greedy thieves almost always leave some piece of evidence at the crime scene — plucked feathers, hair in the wire, or (horror!) headless corpses. You sadly examine the body (or bodies) and find — nothing. What happened?

Immediately call your state veterinarian to report sudden, unexplained high mortality in a flock of chickens. The sudden death of a large portion of the flock can be a sign of deadly, incredibly contagious strains of avian influenza or Newcastle disease. The good news:These diseases aren't present in the United States at this time. If one of those diseases somehow comes into the country and an outbreak occurs, many birds can suffer and die, unless the disease is identified quickly and controlled.

In Table 10-4, we take a stab at summarizing some of the reasons you may find a chicken (that looked fine yesterday) suddenly dead. Many of the diseases on the list can hit a chicken so hard that the bird doesn't have time to show signs of illness. Refer to the Chapters 11 through 14 for detailed information about specific diseases. Read on for a discussion of the special circumstances for sudden death in chicks, growing chickens, and adult chickens.

Table 10-4	Causes of Sudden Death in Chickens		
Type of Disease	**Common Causes**	**Not-So-Common Causes**	**Rare Causes**
Accidents of flock management (see Chapter 11)	Botulism Heat stress Water deprivation	Mold toxins in feed Pesticide toxicity	Carbon monoxide poisoning Medication toxicity PTFE poisoning Shatterproof heat lamps in brooders.
Bacteria or viruses (see Chapter 12)	Colibacillosis	Erysipelas Fowl cholera	Deadly strains of avian influenza and Newcastle disease
Parasites (see Chapter 13)	Coccidiosis	Severe poultry mite infestation	Blackhead

If you encounter any dead chickens, immediately remove them from your flock's environment! Chickens have no taboo against cannibalism, and they will consume dead flock mates. Through this disgusting route, a toxin or infection can spread rapidly through a flock. In particular, botulism can wipe out most of a flock through chickens eating dead chickens or eating the maggots (treats for chickens!) feasting on decomposing carcasses. We give advice on proper carcass disposal in Chapter 18.

Identifying what causes sudden death in chicks

When you have chicks in your flock suddenly die, you have a couple other circumstances to investigate. To the list in Table 10-4, we need to add a few special circumstances of sudden death that are unique to a chicken's first few weeks of life.

- ✓ **Omphalitis:** This is an infection of the belly button. The infection can travel throughout the chick's body so quickly that you may not have any warning of the problem prior to the chick's sudden death. See Chapter 9 for more information.

- ✓ **Hypothermia:** A chick can't regulate its own body temperature for the first two weeks after hatching and needs to be kept warm by momma hen or an artificial heat source. In cold weather, baby chicks without a heat source will quickly die.

Unfortunately, brooder accidents involving heat lamps and poor ventilation are common explanations for when a high proportion of a group of chicks suddenly dies. You can prevent these accidents from happening by adhering to these suggestions:

✔ Make sure that chicks have room to get away from a heat source and avoid overheating. Don't place feed or water dishes directly under the heat source.

✔ Don't use shatterproof versions of heat lamp bulbs, which are usually coated with a substance (PTFE) that can emit a bird-killing gas when overheated.

✔ If you use a fuel-burning heat source in a brooder area, such as a propane heater, make sure you have good ventilation to prevent build-up of carbon dioxide gas. Also, combustion heaters that aren't working properly can emit carbon monoxide, which is deadly to people, chicks, or any other creature that breathes. Installing a carbon monoxide alarm in the brooder area is simple, inexpensive, and possibly life-saving.

Knowing what causes sudden death in growing chickens

Coccidiosis is, by far, the most common infectious cause of death for growing chickens. Coccidia parasites and chickens are insepa-rable; the parasites are found wherever chickens are raised. Although coccidiosis usually gives some warning of its presence in the flock, causing droopiness, weight loss, and bloody droppings, some strains of the parasite can quickly kill an infected chicken. Medications are available to prevent and treat coccidiosis. (Refer to Chapter 13 and the appendix for a list and more information.)

If you've experienced the sudden death of a young chicken, you may have done some research and come across the term *sudden death syndrome* of young meat-type birds. You may be raising the white commercial meat-type chickens in your backyard, and in that case, you should put this mysterious disease on your list of possibilities. More than likely though, you keep dual-purpose heritage breed chickens. Broiler chicken diseases, such as sudden death syndrome, hypoglycemic-spiking mortality syndrome, and heart attacks haven't been confirmed in heritage breed backyard chickens, as far as we know.

Identifying what causes sudden death in adult chickens

Chickens, particularly adult hens, are tough animals. We've been shocked by the severe disease we've seen while looking at the insides of chickens that were "fine one day, and dead the next," according to the flock keeper's observation. Here are a few of the most common rapidly fatal ailments of older hens:

- ✔ **Egg peritonitis:** This is a common cause of death in hens that may sneak up both on the hen and the flock keeper. (We discuss it in Chapter 12.)

- ✔ **Tumors in the abdomen:** Tumors, especially ovarian tumors, are an extremely common cause of sudden death in hens 3 years of age and older.

- ✔ **Fatty liver hemorrhagic syndrome:** This disease abruptly kills the best hen in the flock. She's the pretty, fat hen who lays lots of eggs. See Chapter 11 for more information about this serious problem of spoiled hens.

- ✔ **Nutritional exhaustion:** A hen who has been fed a diet deficient in calcium, phosphorus, vitamin D3, or potassium can die suddenly from nutritional exhaustion. Her body may appear to be in good condition, with an egg in the oviduct ready to be laid.

Overfeeding table scraps or treats to a hard-working hen can unbalance her diet and eventually exhaust her in a nutritional sense. Feed a complete commercial layer diet and restrict the treats. During periods of high egg production in a layer flock, offer oyster shell as a calcium supplement and insurance against deficiency.

Letting the pros figure out the reason for sudden death

Without getting professional help, the cause of death is likely to remain a mystery to you. Don't wait too long to get help, because the internal organs of a bird carcass break down rapidly, erasing clues to the disease. Your best shot at getting a diagnosis is by submitting the bird or birds right away to a veterinary diagnostic lab; we provide tips on submitting good specimens in Chapter 15.

If you can't immediately take a carcass to a laboratory, double-bag and refrigerate it or place the carcass in a cooler with ice. Call your lab to discuss the best way to preserve specimens until you can get them to the lab, so that they'll be in good shape and useful for analysis when they arrive.

Taking a dead bird to a diagnostic laboratory may not be an option for you. In that case, you can perform a postmortem yourself, and possibly find some clues on the inside. It's not difficult; we guide you through a chicken postmortem in Chapter 15.

Part III

A Close-Up Examination of Chicken Woes and Diseases

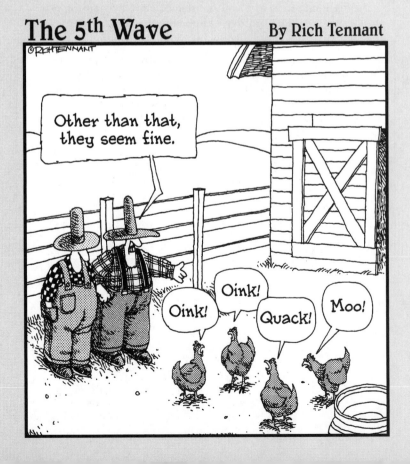

The 5th Wave   By Rich Tennant

Other than that, they seem fine.

Oink!

Oink!

Quack!

Moo!

In this part...

We suspect that you receive advice (whether you ask for it or not) from a variety of sources: friends, the Internet, the guy at the feed store, or an extension agent, to name a few possible chicken health advisors. Maybe a professional, such as a veterinarian or a poultry pathologist at a diagnostic laboratory has given you a specific disease diagnosis.

After you've jotted down the ominous-sounding veterinary jargon that your advice-giver mentioned, we bet you have a lot more questions. In this part, we help you understand more about the major chicken diseases, briefing you on the cause, the signs and means of spread, prevention tips, and treatment advice.

Chapter 11

Accidents of Flock Management

● ●

In This Chapter

▶ Defending against assaults by airborne and ground-based predators

▶ Psychoanalyzing feather peckers and cannibal hens

▶ Correcting nutrient excesses and deficiencies

▶ Avoiding poisons — natural and synthetic

▶ Spotting dangers in and out of the chicken coop

● ●

*T*he diseases we cover in this chapter aren't caused by germs or worms, but by bad luck, extreme weather, and human error. We put them roughly in order of importance for backyard flocks. Predators are the number one cause of death for backyard poultry, and bodily harm by bullying hens isn't far behind.

You, the flock keeper, may not be at fault for nutritional disorders, toxicities, or environmental stresses, but management mistakes can certainly make these problems much worse. We review the causes and effects of the problems and give some advice on diagnosis and prevention. If treatment is an option, we mention that, too.

Identifying and Defending Against Predators

You can say that this section is the most important in this book, because predators are by far the leading cause of death for backyard poultry. Believing that you must know your enemy in order to defeat your enemy, we present the criminal profiles of North American serial chicken killers in Table 11-1.

Table 11-1	Profiles of Chicken Killers	
Pattern	*Time of Day*	*Possible Culprits*
One missing bird	Day	Dog, hawk
	Night	Coyote, fox, owl
Many missing birds	Night	Fox
Missing heads	Day	Hawk
	Night	Raccoon, owl
Missing eggs	Day	Rat, snake
	Night	Fox, opossum, rat, skunk, weasel
Many scattered carcasses	Day	Dog
	Night	Coyote, weasel
Chicks missing or eaten	Day	Cat, hawk
	Night	Skunk
Birds with missing feathers and small wounds	Day or night	Cat
Layers with wounds in the vent area	Day	Other chickens
Missing limbs	Night	Raccoon
Vent area eaten	Night	Opossum, weasel
Carcass buried in leaves and dirt	Day or night	Bobcat, fox

Predators almost always work unobserved. If you stumble across a predator's crime scene and find an animal with the carcass, keep in mind that the animal may not be the guilty party, but only a scavenger cleaning up after the fact. You need to put on your sleuthing cap and investigate to identify the killer. Look for signs on the carcass and around the kill site, such as

- Location of the bite wounds
- Size of the bite wounds
- Perpetrator hair or droppings left at the scene

The best way to keep chickens safe from predators is to keep them indoors all the time, but that's not compatible with the free-range lifestyle that backyard chickens (and flock keepers) prefer. Chickens can figure out how to be predator-savvy during the day, but they're completely vulnerable at night. Unless you intend to provide a buffet for the neighborhood carnivores, you must lock chickens up at night in a predator-proof building. Read on for ideas about keeping backyard chickens safe.

The air attack: Possible countermeasures

Two categories of defense measures are useful for warding off hawks, owls, and other predatory birds: barriers and scare tactics.

 Birds of prey most often use the hunting technique of perching high to scan the terrain and size up their prey. The hunting bird launches from the perch to swoop down onto its chosen victim. If you put up a barrier to the "swoop zone," an aerial hunter may choose an easier flight path somewhere else. Here are some ideas for barriers:

- ✔ **Cover the top of the chicken pen with netting.** You can find plastic bird netting at lawn and garden stores, or *flight pen netting* is available from poultry supply companies.

- ✔ **Suspend a grid of wires or string above the pen.** You can use nylon fishing line, stainless steel wire, or string for the grid lines. Space the lines 2 to 3 feet apart. Step-in posts found at farm stores are useful for holding up grid lines in moveable pens or in open spaces that lack fences or trees to tie the lines to. Make the grid lines extra scary by tying a streamer of shiny bird-deterrent tape to them every few feet.

- ✔ **Provide hawk-raid shelters for chickens to duck into.** A hideout can be simple, such as a cave made of straw bales. Natural cover like bushes and trees is potential shelter, too.

 Scare tactics work best when you combine several methods and mix them up every once in a while. You have to keep bird predators on their toes, or they'll become bored and ignore your efforts. Select from this bag of tricks:

- ✔ **Put up a scarecrow.** A scarecrow is most effective if it appears to move. Change the scarecrow's position every few days and use your creativity to make it move in the breeze, perhaps with pinwheels or flags.

✔ **Hang shiny things from strings.** Items, such as aluminum pie pans or discarded compact discs that move and flash in a breeze, work well.

✔ **Place a cheap mirror, facing upward, in the bottom of an empty hanging plant basket.** Hang several of these baskets around the pen or coop. A mirror flashes in the sunlight and makes birds of prey suspect danger.

✔ **Add a flood light or strobe light.** A motion-activated light scares off owls.

✔ **Fight fire with fire.** Encourage a *kestrel,* also known as a *sparrow hawk,* to move into your neighborhood by putting up kestrel nest boxes. The American kestrel is a small bird of prey found in most areas of North and South America that prefers to eat grasshoppers and rodents, not chickens. Kestrels aggressively defend their territory from larger hawks, harassing the bigger birds until they're driven off. You can find plans online to build and properly place nest boxes that are inviting homes for kestrels.

Don't even think about killing a bird of prey. Birds of prey in the United States are protected by the Migratory Bird Treaty Act and by state and tribal laws. Killing a hawk or owl is punishable by hefty fines and possibly jail time.

The ground assault: Possible countermeasures

Four-legged predators are a problem for every flock keeper, even in urban and suburban environments. Some flock keepers manage to keep birds alive in areas where predator pressure from coyotes, dogs, raccoons, and opossums is ridiculously high.

You can train your chickens to put themselves to bed inside a predator-proof coop at dusk. Shoo them into the coop every evening at dusk for a week or two, and they'll start following the routine on their own. When closed up for the night, a predator-proof coop shouldn't have any opening larger than 1 x 1 inch. Consider these other bits of advice:

✔ **Avoid so-called "chicken wire" when you build your secure nighttime coop.** We think chicken wire should be renamed "raccoon snack wire," because the gaps in that style of fencing are perfectly spaced for nimble raccoon fingers to reach through and grab the necks of sleeping chickens.

✔ **Lay down a 2-foot-wide apron of wire fencing along the base of a fence or pen.** You can bury the wire, or simply lay it on the ground, pinning it down with rocks, bricks, or stakes. Doing so can keep predators from digging underneath. Okay, here's a good use for chicken wire.

✔ **Build your coops on stilts.** They discourage snakes and rodents from getting inside.

✔ **Use electrified poultry netting.** Electricity is extremely effective against any critter with paws and a wet nose. We're big fans of electric poultry netting. If you properly set it up, it works very well to keep birds in and predators out.

Building an electric fence is cheap and easy compared to installing other types of fencing. Many online resources for do-it-yourself electric fence construction are available, and you can also get advice from staff at farm-supply stores. The keys to an effective electric fence are a powerful, *low-impedance* fence charger and good electrical grounding. Buy a fence charger that's much bigger than you think you need (you almost can't overdo it) and don't skimp on ground rods.

Addressing Flock-Mate Persecution or Cannibalism

Flock-mate persecution is a serious behavior problem that can affect all types of chicken flocks: commercial or backyard, caged or free- range, organic or conventional. Researchers have extensively studied the phenomenon of persecution in chicken flocks, but they still have many unanswered questions about why it happens, or what you can do to prevent it. For whatever reason, chickens may peck at a flock mate's vent, feathers, or other parts of the body so badly that they create serious wounds, even causing her death. Flock keepers call this extreme form of persecution *cannibalism,* because chickens actually devour the flesh of flock mates.

These sections take a closer look at the types of persecution behaviors (including cannibalism) that you may see in your flock and how to prevent or limit them as much as possible.

Noticing persecution behavior

You can spot flock behavior problems if you spend daily quality time observing your chickens. Here are two common forms of persecution behavior problems to watch out for:

✔ **Feather pecking:** Dominant birds peck at birds further down the pecking order, often plucking out feathers, or in severe cases, causing bleeding wounds that attract more pecking from other flock mates. The appearance of blood on exposed skin may stir the flock into a frenzy of pecking at the victim, who can die from her injuries. This extreme form of flock-mate persecution is often called cannibalism.

✔ **Vent pecking:** This behavior seems to be separate from feather pecking, although both problems can appear in the same flock. It usually happens soon after hens start an egg-laying period, so it may be linked to hormonal changes. Vent pecking is more commonly seen in *floor-layers* (hens that choose to lay their eggs on the floor instead of a nest) living in crowded conditions. Just after laying an egg, a hen's cloaca tissue protrudes a little bit from the vent, and the exposed red membranes attract attention and pecking from other birds. As with feather pecking, vent pecking can escalate into a frenzy in which the victim can be seriously injured, even disemboweled by the aggressors.

Why do chickens commit these acts of violence? No one is completely sure. A combination of factors are probably at work, including boredom, hormone surges, personality disorders, or nutrition. Chickens need to forage and explore their environment with their beaks; persecution is likely to be normal foraging and pecking behavior gone horribly wrong.

Taking action to prevent or correct these behaviors

You can't predict outbreaks of persecution; they unfortunately can happen even when flock keepers take preventive or corrective measures. After the persecution habit starts, other members of the flock quickly learn it, and it's extremely difficult to break. We list some preventive and corrective measures here, because they're helpful in many cases, especially when you combine several methods.

Housing suggestions

You can design your flock's living space in a way that keeps chickens engaged in nondestructive behavior, instead of pecking at each other, using the following suggestions:

✔ **Avoid overcrowding.** Measure the size of your flock's living space and compare it to the minimum space allowances we suggest in Chapter 5.

✔ **Provide at least one nest box for every five hens.** Mount the nest boxes no higher than 18 inches off the ground.

✔ **Provide escape sanctuaries for persecuted birds.** They can include a natural cover from bushes, straw bale caves, a dog house, or a pet carrier.

✔ **Hang up toys in the coop to distract and redirect pecking behavior.** Some dangling toys that seem to keep chickens' interest are white ropes, aluminum pie plates, compact discs, or a head of cabbage.

Nutrition suggestions

Not only do chickens require certain nutrients to stay physically healthy, but they also need a daily allowance of pecking in order to stay mentally healthy. You can feed your flock in a way that provides for both mental and physical needs. Consider these tips:

✔ **Feed a complete commercial layer diet in mash form, rather than pellets.** Chickens spend more time eating a meal of fine mash particles than pellets, so it keeps them occupied longer with constructive pecking.

✔ **Feed "keep them busy" high-fiber treats in late afternoon, when feather pecking incidents peak.** Hay, greens, or vegetable scraps that require disassembly (watermelon rinds or smashed pumpkins come to mind) are good choices. Compressed blocks of grains — also known as *peck blocks* — are also helpful diversions that are available at most feed stores.

✔ **Include a little animal protein in the diet.** Mealworms, black soldier grubs, farmed worms, or an occasional handful of cat food may satisfy cravings for meat.

Medical and management advice

Preventing persecution with the previous housing and nutrition ideas is much more successful than correcting the behavior after the flock starts tearing into each other. If your prevention efforts fail and flock mates are waging war in the coop, here's what you can do to treat the injured and restore peace:

✔ **Consider fashion eyewear.** You can fit repeat offenders with plastic blinders (also called *peepers* or *chicken spectacles*) that are secured to the beak with a clip in the nostrils. Bespectacled chickens can forage, eat, and drink, but they can't attack their flock mates. See Chapter 17 for more information about the pros and cons of peepers and how to install them.

✔ **Spray plucked patches with anti-peck spray or pine tar.** Doing so can discourage further pecking.

✓ **Separate an injured bird from the rest of the flock until her wounds heal.** We describe a hospital cage where you can isolate and nurse injured birds in Chapter 17.

✓ **Avoid keeping persecution ringleaders for breeding purposes, because aggression to some extent may be an inherited trait.** How do you identify the instigators? They're the ones with perfect plumage, when every other bird in the flock has a bare butt or plucked head. For the flock's sake, you may judge that the death penalty is appropriate for a repeat offender and *cull* (euthanize or slaughter) the bird.

Eyeing Nutritional Disorders

Nutritional disorders are unusual in backyard flocks fed complete commercial poultry diets appropriate for the birds' stages of life. Old feed, poorly balanced homemade diets, and feeding an excessive number of treats are the most common reasons for nutritional blunders.

Problems from unbalanced diets don't happen overnight; these problems of nutrient excesses or deficiencies take weeks to months for signs to appear in a flock. You can fix many nutritional problems if you catch them early. These sections help you identify the chickens in your flock who may suffer from nutritional disorders.

Not just fluffy: Obesity

A big, fluffy hen is an appealing sight, but when she's not just fluffy, but fat — then you have a health problem on your hands. Fat hens are generally less fertile and lay fewer eggs than their flock mates of average size. Obesity may lead to liver and kidney disorders in both hens and roosters and predispose hens to serious malfunctions of the reproductive system, such as peritonitis or vent prolapse.

A common consequence of obesity in older backyard hens is *fatty liver hemorrhagic syndrome*. Fat is deposited in the liver of an obese hen, making the liver tissue soft, fragile, and prone to bleeding. When an affected hen strains to lay an egg, her fatty liver can actually fall apart, and the hen will quickly bleed to death.

Fluffy feathers disguise a chicken's body condition, so you may not notice how big she's getting unless you feel her breastbone and find a layer of fat and bulging breast muscles. We describe how to measure body condition in Chapter 7.

The bossy hen at the top of the pecking order is more likely than her flock mates to be overweight. She aggressively ensures that she's first to get her fair share (plus) at meal time. High-energy diets, particularly unbalanced homemade diets that are mostly corn or only scratch feed, encourage obesity in backyard flocks.

Flock keepers have been known to kill their birds with kindness by overfeeding sugary baked goods and other high-energy treats. If you find that your big hen isn't just fluffy, but fat, then you need to cut the carbs. Stick to a commercial layer diet and eliminate treats, scratch feed, and corn.

During their waking hours, hens should always have a complete balanced layer diet available. We don't ever recommend feed restriction for hard-working laying hens.

Excess calcium

Diets for laying hens contain a lot of calcium in order to meet hens' enormous need for calcium to produce lots of eggs with strong shells. Layer diets contain roughly three times the amount of calcium that non-laying chickens need. (Refer to Chapter 6 for what a layer diet means for your hens.)

If you feed young chickens diets meant for layers for several weeks, the excess dietary calcium can wreck their kidneys and create kidney stones. The damage from excess calcium remains even after pullets grow up and begin to lay eggs; in general, they have a shorter, less-productive lifespan. Don't feed layer diets to growing chickens. You can switch to layer feed when pullets are 4 months old to prepare them nutritionally for egg-laying.

Vitamin and mineral deficiencies

The most common reason for vitamin and mineral deficiencies to show up in a flock is a mistake in preparing the feed, whether the feed was mixed at home or at a commercial feed mill. In other words, someone forgot to add the vitamin-mineral premix. Old, stale feed and antibiotic use are less-common causes of vitamin deficiencies. Vitamins can break down over time or with high temperature and humidity, so feed that's been stored for longer than two months may lose nutritional value. Antibiotic use can interfere with a body's ability to absorb vitamins and minerals.

When you feed chickens diets that lack vitamins or minerals for weeks to months, signs of B-vitamin deficiencies usually show up first; signs of other vitamin and mineral deficiencies take longer to appear. Table 11-2 shows major vitamin and mineral deficiencies and the common signs they cause in chickens.

Table 11-2	Chicken Vitamin and Mineral Deficiency Syndromes	
Deficiency	*Signs in Growing Birds*	*Signs in Adult Chickens*
B vitamins	Poor hatches, stunted growth, poor feathering, limping, curled toes	Decreased egg production
Vitamin A	Watery or cheesy white discharge from the eyes, staggering, stunted growth	Decreased egg production, wasting
Calcium and vitamin D3	Rickets (stunted growth, limping, rubbery beak and toes, twisted keel)	Thin-shelled eggs, broken bones, sudden death
Vitamin E	Crazy chick disease (no coordination, tremors, twisted neck)	No outward signs of deficiency
Vitamin K	Bleeding or severe bruising from minor wounds, poor hatches	Bleeding or severe bruising from minor wounds
Manganese, along with other nutrients	Perosis (slipped tendon, leg deformity)	Thin-shelled eggs

Correcting the diet is the long-term fix for nutritional disorders. For emergency treatment, add a poultry vitamin and mineral supplement, available from feed stores or poultry-supply companies, to the drinking water according to label directions. Provide the fortified water as the flock's only source of drinking water for two weeks.

Recognizing Sources of Poisonings in Your Backyard

Everything is toxic, even water, oxygen, salt, and all nutrients; it's just a matter of dose. In this section we cover the toxic events most likely to happen to backyard poultry and explain how you can avoid them.

Botulism

Chickens get *botulism* by eating food or drinking water containing *botulinum toxin,* which is produced by *Clostridium botulinum* bacteria. We use the word *food* loosely here, because chickens are most frequently poisoned with botulism by eating dead flock mates or the fly larvae that have been feasting on chicken carcasses. Botulism bacteria are commonly found in soil, and they thrive in warm, wet environments with rotting vegetation, spoiled food, or decomposing carcasses.

Botulinum toxins are the most potent toxins known; only tiny doses are needed to paralyze the nervous system and kill an affected bird. Sick chickens, if you discover them still alive, will usually be sitting on the ground, hunched over, and unable to stand or hold their heads up. Botulism causes floppy paralysis of the legs, wings, and neck, an effect which gives the disease another name, *limberneck.* Often, chickens are found dead, with no signs of a struggle.

Several types of botulinum toxin exist, and some, but not all botulinum toxin types can poison people. The type of botulinum toxin that usually causes disease in poultry (type C) doesn't affect people.

 Diagnosing botulism can be difficult with laboratory tests, but a diagnostic laboratory can try. You should suspect botulism if several (maybe many) chickens in a flock are suddenly struck by floppy paralysis. Affected birds are often the largest, healthiest, and more dominant members of the flock, because they're likely to push away low-status birds from the contaminated food and hog it for themselves.

 You can prevent botulism outbreaks by picking up and disposing of animal carcasses immediately, including mice and frogs. Don't feed spoiled human food, especially home-canned vegetables. Don't let chickens have access to drying-up ponds in the summertime, because the bacteria love warm, wet, rotting vegetation and decomposing aquatic creatures.

No specific treatment for botulism is available to backyard flock keepers. You can attempt to flush some of the toxin out of the birds' systems with a laxative solution (see the appendix). Some birds will recover if they're isolated and given good nursing care for several days to several weeks; it's a waiting game.

Household poisons

You can safely assume household chemicals that are toxic to people or pets are also toxic to chickens. Insecticides, rat poison, antifreeze, fertilizer, and mothballs can poison poultry.

Chickens are frequently poisoned by good intentions when flock keepers spray birds with house and garden insecticides to kill poultry lice or mites. Hence, you should only use products labeled for use on chickens and should follow those label directions precisely. Veterinarians can also prescribe safe and effective external parasite treatments for chickens and give you an egg discard time.

If you think your chicken may have been poisoned by a chemical kept around the house or applied to the yard, follow these simple steps:

1. **Get rid of the suspected toxin right away, or put the bird and her flock mates in an uncontaminated place.**

2. **Call the Animal Poison Control Center at 888-426-4435 or contact an avian veterinarian.**

   Human poison control centers are unlikely to be able to give bird-specific advice.

If you accidentally spill oil products or other chemicals on a chicken's feathers or skin, make sure you promptly remove them with a bath of warm water and liquid dish detergent, followed by plenty of rinsing with warm water.

Lead poisoning

Birds are very susceptible to lead poisoning because ingested lead objects tend to lodge in the gizzard, where they're ground and slowly absorbed. Potential sources of lead in a chicken's environment include the following: shotgun pellets, fishing weights, batteries, paint chips, and contaminated dirt. Lead poisoning in poultry is a human health concern, because significant amounts of lead can be found in the meat and eggs of lead-exposed chickens.

Chickens suffering from lead poisoning become thin and weak and may have nervous system signs, such as lack of coordination, limping, or paralysis. A veterinarian or diagnostic laboratory can diagnose lead poisoning by taking a blood test or by measuring lead in organ tissue.

Scout your flock's environment and remove loose metal objects and sources of peeling paint. The foundations of old buildings aren't good foraging ground for chickens, because lead paint scrapings accumulated over the years may have contaminated the soil.

Treating lead poisoning isn't a do-it-yourself job. Avian veterinarians can treat lead poisoning in pet birds with long-term lead-binding medications. Don't use meat or eggs (either for eating or hatching) from chickens that are exposed to lead or treated for lead poisoning for meat or eggs.

Mold toxins in feed (Mycotoxins)

A *mycotoxin* is a toxic substance produced naturally by a fungus (mold). Some fungi like to grow on grain and other feed ingredients but may not be visible as obvious mold growth. Scientists have discovered hundreds of mycotoxins, and many of them make chickens sick when they eat contaminated grains or processed feed. You can notice a wide range of signs in poultry poisoned by mycotoxins, including decreased appetite and egg production, poor growth and feathering, and crusty sores on the skin, beak, toes, or inside of the mouth. Mycotoxins can also cause sudden death of poultry.

Diagnosing mycotoxin poisoning is a challenge because the signs mimic so many other diseases, and because only specialized laboratories perform testing for mycotoxins in feed. You may suspect mycotoxin poisoning when you notice that an onset of a problem coincides with feeding a new batch or type of feed.

To prevent poisonings connected with toxic mold, purchase commercial pelleted or crumbled diets. The process of making pelleted or crumbled feed destroys some fungal spores. Feed manufacturers routinely conduct tests for mycotoxins in the raw ingredients that go into commercial feed and reject ingredients or recall products that are found to be contaminated.

To further prevent the chance of your flock being affected by mycotoxins, you can store feed in a cool, dry location for no more than two months. Don't feed your flock moldy stuff. Periodically empty feeders and feed bins, remove old feed stuck to crevices, and clean and disinfect as a final step (see Chapter 5).

Treatment consists of removing the toxic feed and replacing it with mycotoxin-free stuff. Chickens usually recover quickly after uncontaminated feed is provided.

Toxic gas

Overheated nonstick cookware emits a gas that's deadly poisonous to birds. We're not making it up. Polytetrafluoroethylene (PTFE) is the name of the nonstick coating that breaks down and forms a gas when heated past about 500 degrees Fahrenheit (260 degrees Celsius). The gas destroys lung and liver tissue of birds, but doesn't appear to harm people or other animals. Birds are killed so quickly that even if treatment were available (no known treatment is available), you wouldn't have time to react.

PTFE poisoning is a concern for flock keepers who brood their chicks in the kitchen or have house-pet chickens (not as uncommon as you may think). In addition to nonstick cookware, the high-temperature self-cleaning cycle of some ovens can release the gas, because oven interiors may have a nonstick coating. If you keep birds in the house, get ready to scrub more and ban the nonstick pans and self-clean oven cycle, to stay on the safe side.

Don't use shatterproof versions of heat-lamp bulbs to keep chickens warm. PTFE coating on the bulb is what makes it shatterproof. Chicks have died from exposure to gas emitted by this style of heat-lamp bulb. (Refer to Chapter 5 for more information about heat-lamp bulbs.)

Toxic foods and plants

Although flock keepers worry about the crazy things chickens may eat (what's the deal with the craving for packing peanuts?), cases of chickens being poisoned by table scraps and yard plants are uncommon, as we explain in these sections.

Table scraps

Warnings about toxic table scraps are mostly myths. In general, if you can eat it, your chickens can, too, but moderation is the key when recycling table scraps to feed a backyard flock. Bingeing on alcohol, chocolate, or any food isn't good for anyone or any bird. Even avocado toxicity, which has been reported in canaries, budgerigars, and ostriches (but not chickens as far as we know), is a matter of overindulgence, and mucho guacamole is easily avoided.

Our advice is to keep it simple:

- ✔ If you wouldn't eat it, don't feed it to your chickens.
- ✔ Don't feed any treat in large quantities.

Toxic plants

Many types of plants make noxious substances that discourage herbivores from eating them into extinction. In large enough doses, these natural plant-eater deterrents can have toxic effects on your flock.

Much of what scientists think they know about toxic plants for poultry is borrowed from reports of human, livestock, and pet toxicities, but in reality, they're mostly guessing. Scientists don't know much about the types and doses of plant toxins that affect free-range chickens. Fortunately, plant poisonings are very rare occurrences in chicken flocks, perhaps because chickens possess some instinctive nutritional wisdom. If they have a choice, they'll reject a food that tastes funny to them.

Hungry chickens, however, are much more likely to consume toxic plants than well-fed chickens; eating bad weeds is better than eating nothing at all, we suppose. Make sure your pastured poultry always have good pasture available. If not, move the flock to fresh ground with plenty of foraging choices.

Identifying Housing and Environmental Dangers

In Chapter 5, we discuss ways to keep the flock clean and comfortable. If something goes terribly wrong with those efforts, the diseases we list in this section can be the result. Unfortunately, in many cases of housing or environmental disasters, treatment of the affected birds is too late to be successful, although using preventive measures for the rest of the flock is never too late.

Frostbite

Chickens can tolerate cold weather, and they can tolerate wet conditions, but the combination of wet and below-freezing temperatures is a recipe for frostbite.

Combs, wattles, and toes are susceptible to frostbite. The first sign of frostbite is swelling of the affected part, usually within 24 hours of the cold injury. Also early on, frostbitten combs and wattles may blister and leak clear fluid, but frostbitten chicken toes don't form blisters. It will take weeks to see the full extent of the damage, but a visible line eventually will separate the healthy tissue closer to the body from the damaged tissue farther out. The damaged parts will gradually turn black, and they usually fall off.

Frostbite is very painful. A rooster may not want to eat because his sore, frostbitten wattles bump into the feeder.

Keep the coop dry and block the wind to prevent frostbite. Some flock keepers swear by a coating of petroleum jelly to protect combs and wattles on cold nights. If you live in a cold climate, choose chicken breeds with small facial appendages.

Taking cues from treatment of human victims of frostbite, we can point out a few things that may help frostbitten chickens and a few that do more harm than good.

Do the following for frostbite:

- ✓ **Apply a dab of aloe vera ointment to the affected area daily.** You can find aloe vera ointment at most pharmacies.

- ✓ **Administer anti-inflammatory medications that your veterinarian prescribes.** If a veterinarian isn't available, an aspirin solution can be used (see the appendix).

Don't do the following for frostbite:

- ✓ **Don't massage the affected parts.** Massaging adds to the tissue damage.

- ✓ **Don't be in a rush to trim off black, dead tissue.** It takes a while to know how far the damage goes, and often the dead tissue eventually falls off on its own. As a gruesome old medical adage says, "Frostbitten in January, amputate in July."

Hardware disease

Free-range poultry are at risk of picking up and eating small metal objects as they forage. Why they eat these things, we don't know. Coins, tacks, wire, and screws are commonly found in the gizzards of birds that have died of *hardware disease.* The metal objects cause damage, and eventually death, by irritating the gizzard's lining, by blocking the passage of food, or in the worst-case scenario, by piercing through the gizzard and setting up a fatal infection in the abdomen.

Hardware disease is rarely recognized prior to the affected chicken's death, although a veterinarian can diagnose it with X-rays. Even if you discover hardware disease in a live bird, treatment isn't typically successful because gizzard surgery is very risky. In hindsight, a flock keeper may recall that the affected bird had a poor appetite, lost weight, and seemed in pain.

 To prevent hardware disease, get the junk pile out of the chicken pen. Regularly check the area for bits of metal. We suggest you use a construction site clean-up magnet, which is available at hardware stores, for screening chicken runs for metal objects. Don't bed the coop with wood shavings donated by carpenters or woodworkers, because the material often has screws, nails, or other hardware inadvertently mixed in.

Heat stress

All chickens suffer in hot and humid weather, but adult chickens really have a hard time coping. Egg production drops among

heat-stressed hens, and their eggs may be thin-shelled. Flock fertility declines because roosters don't feel like going to work. Because
chickens don't feel like eating in hot weather either, young birds
grow more slowly.

 When temperatures climb above 85 degrees Fahrenheit (29 degrees
Celsius), chickens pant and hold their wings away from their bodies
to cool off. The situation becomes serious when the mercury hits
100 degrees F (38 degrees C) and higher; birds may become listless and die of heat stress. Emergency cooling measures, such as
shade, fans, and plenty of cool drinking water, are necessary for
survival.

 In addition to the cooling-off tips we provide in Chapter 5, you can
treat birds suffering from heat stress with a vitamin and electrolyte
supplement in the drinking water. Supplements designed for poultry
are often available at farm supply stores. Vitamin C especially
seems to help birds live through hot spells. If your vitamin and
electrolyte supplement doesn't contain vitamin C (also called
ascorbic acid), you can crush one 1,000 mg vitamin C tablet and
mix it into each gallon of drinking water.

Starve-outs

Occasionally and sadly, a baby chick fails to learn to eat and drink,
eventually dying from starvation and dehydration. That poor chick
is called a *starve-out,* or a *nonstarter.* Starving-out is a rare phenomenon among chicks raised naturally by hens, but it's unfortunately
fairly common for artificially incubated chicks.

Chicks can get off to a bad start for a number of reasons: less than
ideal incubator conditions, chilling, or shipping are a few big ones.
If feeders are difficult to get to, chicks may eat bedding instead
and plug themselves up with indigestible stuff. Chick deaths due to
starving-out usually happen within three to five days after hatch.

 Here are some tips for preventing starve-outs:

   ✔ **Use starter crumbles as bedding for the first two days.**
     Everything the chicks peck at is food.

   ✔ **Keep a light on in the brooder around the clock until the
     chicks have the eating thing down pat.** A heat lamp on all of
     the time serves both heat and light purposes.

   ✔ **Place starter crumbles in shallow trays or cookie sheets in
     the brooder.** That way, the chicks can easily stumble across
     the food.

✔ **Frequently visit the brooder and stir up the chicks.** Doing so encourages them to move around, explore, and eat.

✔ **Let the older chicks be good role models.** You can keep chicks that are a few days older and well-started with the hatchlings to show them the ropes.

Suffocation

Chickens, especially chicks and growing birds, can suffocate each other when birds are crowded or piled in a corner. *Piling* is common when birds are moved to a new place, when they're frightened, or when chicks are cold. Deaths due to suffocation happen more frequently at night.

You can prevent suffocation deaths by following these tips:

✔ **Eliminate corners.** Use corrugated cardboard brooder guard to form a circular pen for chicks.

✔ **Leave a nightlight or other dim light in the brooder or coop for new birds the first few nights after bringing them home.** They'll be less frightened and less likely to crowd together for security if they have a nightlight.

✔ **Frequently check new birds.** Make sure you check them late in the evening to ensure they're not piling on each other.

Chapter 12

My Chicken Has What? Diseases Caused by Bacteria and Viruses

. . . .

In This Chapter

▶ Preventing and treating chicken bacterial infections

▶ Thwarting hijacking attempts by chicken viruses

. . . .

*T*his chapter is intended as a resource to answer your questions about the infectious chicken diseases that bacteria or viruses cause. The infections we list here are the ones more likely to affect backyard chickens, or to cause worry for flock keepers. First, we provide a brief dossier of each of the major chicken bacterial infections, and then we do the same for the viral infections, listing them in alphabetical order for easy reference. We give you the highlights of what we suspect you really want to know: the cause and signs of the disease, the prognosis, and hints on prevention and treatment.

If your chickens are healthy at the moment, and we hope they are, we don't recommend that you read this encyclopedic list of woes in its entirety right now or try to memorize the material. We want you to know the information is here when you need it, which may be when your veterinarian, veterinary diagnostic laboratory, or fellow flock keeper suggests that your chicken may be suffering from one of these maladies.

Flock Keeper Beware: Infectious Diseases Caused by Bacteria

Bacteria are everywhere, and mostly they mind their own business, harming no one. Some of these simple organisms are actually beneficial to larger creatures, such as chickens, that they live on or in. The bad guys of the bacterial world are rare, but when they're bad, they're deadly. Here we identify some of the bad bacteria that cause concern for flock keepers everywhere, either because they're common, troublesome to eradicate, or deadly for chickens. Each disease dossier gives you a place to start when you need to research a diagnosis you've been given for your chicken.

Avian intestinal spirochetosis

Spirochetes are long, thin, spring-shaped bacteria that are the cause of *avian intestinal spirochetosis (AIS)*. The spirochetes infect the lining of the cecum and lower intestine of chickens, causing diarrhea and decreased egg production in hens.

If you notice diarrhea-stained eggshells, your flock may be infected with AIS. Because AIS is difficult to diagnose, diagnostic laboratories don't routinely look for it. However, surveys suggest that it's probably much more common than veterinarians realize, especially in free-range hens. Certain strains of AIS spirochetes are also known to occasionally infect people.

Some good news: You can prevent the infection by raising hens off the ground in wire-floored cages, but we're sure that's not a welcome suggestion for backyard flock keepers. Because wild ducks and geese can carry AIS spirochetes, keeping them out of your hens' living space is a good idea.

Antibiotics tilmicosin and lincomycin treat AIS effectively, but because these drugs aren't approved for use in treating laying hens in the United States, you should talk to your veterinarian about AIS treatment options.

Avian tuberculosis

Avian tuberculosis, called *avian TB* for short, is a contagious disease of birds caused by *Mycobacterium avium,* a bacterial organism that is closely related to the one that causes human tuberculosis. In fact, people can be infected by the avian TB organism, but they usually contract it from sources other than chickens, such as soil or other people.

Poultry farmers have been aware of avian TB for more than 100 years. These days, the disease is rare in commercial poultry farms, but it still pops up from time to time in backyard flocks, and it can be a serious problem for zoo birds. In the United States, avian TB is more common in the Midwest than in southern or western states.

The disease is usually seen in older birds as a vague ADR (ain't doin' right) syndrome; affected birds are droopy, tire easily, and become very skinny, even though they may have a good appetite. On the inside, birds with TB develop lumps in the sinuses, liver, or intestines. Sick birds usually go downhill slowly and live for several months before dying of the infection.

No practical treatment exists for backyard chickens with avian TB. Sick birds contaminate the soil in their environment with the TB organisms, which are super-durable and can infect chickens for years to come. The wisest course of action to deal with a TB-infected flock is *depopulation* (euthanizing all the birds), abandoning the site, and raising chickens somewhere else.

Colibacillosis (E. coli infections)

Colibacillosis isn't one disease but a group of diseases caused by certain strains of *Escherichia coli* organisms (*E. coli* for short). Inside the intestines of just about every healthy animal is a metropolis of *E. coli* organisms, which are normal and beneficial inhabitants. Only a few rogue strains of *E. coli* are responsible for colibacillosis.

Poultry scientists generally agree that colibacillosis is the most common infectious disease of chickens. Various forms of colibacillosis affect different stages of a chicken's life, causing *omphalitis* (navel infections) in chicks (see Chapter 9), air-sac infections and diarrhea in growing birds, reproductive tract infections in laying hens, and bumblefoot (a foot infection) in adult birds (see Chapter 14).

Infected birds (including wild birds), rodent droppings, contaminated well water, and things contaminated with bird poop can introduce the illness-causing strains of *E. coli* to flocks. Flies and beetles can spread it. Hens can transmit the infection to their chicks through their eggs.

Healthy, happy birds are quite resistant to colibacillosis, but stressed-out flocks and birds sick with another illness are prone to the infection — a double-whammy. Because colibacillosis goes hand in hand with another disease, figuring out which one caused the illness can be difficult.

Sudden death may be the only sign of colibacillosis. Sick birds sit hunched up with ruffled feathers, not caring if you approach or pick them up. They're often persecuted by healthier flock mates, so they may be found huddled under feeders or in corners.

Infection of a hen's reproductive tract with nasty strains of *E. coli* can result in *egg peritonitis,* a very common cause of death of older laying hens in backyard flocks. This disease gets its name from the layer of stuff that looks like cooked egg coating the inside of an infected bird's abdomen. A hen with egg peritonitis stops laying eggs, has a firm, distended abdomen, and may walk like a penguin. She's often mistaken for an egg-bound bird having difficulty laying an egg.

You can prevent colibacillosis from affecting your flock by follow- ing good biosecurity practices and keeping the flock clean, com- fortable, and well fed. See Chapters 4, 5, and 6 for pointers. Select only very clean hatching eggs to put in your incubator.

Colibacillosis has always been difficult to treat, but these days it's even more challenging because many illness-causing strains of *E. coli* have developed resistance to several types of antibiotics. Here are some potential treatments:

✔ Among the antibiotics that are permitted for use in poultry in the United States, tetracycline, lincomycin, spectinomycin, and sulfa drugs are sometimes effective.

✔ Probiotics, oregano, and vitamin E have been tried as organic preventives or treatments for colibacillosis with mixed results.

✔ Using household bleach as a drinking water sanitizer may limit the spread of the infection through the flock's drinking water (see the appendix for the recipe).

Fowl cholera

Fowl cholera is a contagious disease of domestic and wild birds caused by the bacterial organism *Pasteurella multocida.* Chickens older than 4 months are susceptible to infection. Because most chicks in backyard flocks are hatched in the spring, outbreaks of fowl cholera usually happen in the late summer, autumn, and winter when the year's hatchlings have grown up.

After they're infected, birds can carry the infection for life; these carrier birds are the main way that the disease is introduced and perpetuated in flocks. Fowl cholera isn't an egg-transmitted disease.

Sudden death may be the first indication of the disease, or the affected chicken may drool, breathe with difficulty, have diarrhea, and develop a dark-colored comb. Later, if the chicken survives the initial stage, swellings develop in wattles, face, foot pads, leg joints, or wing joints. The mortality rate in an affected flock ranges from 10 to 50 percent.

To prevent introducing fowl cholera to your flock, don't bring home adult birds. Vaccines exist to protect birds against fowl cholera, but they're rarely used in backyard flocks. Treatment of an infected flock with sulfa drugs or tetracycline reduces deaths from fowl cholera but doesn't eliminate the infection.

Infectious coryza

Infectious coryza, also known as *roup* or *cold,* is a respiratory disease of chickens caused by the bacterial organism *Haemophilus paragallinarum.* Carrier chickens, sick or healthy-looking, are the source of infection for backyard flocks. Infectious coryza isn't egg-transmitted.

Here's the usual scenario for an outbreak of infectious coryza in a backyard flock:

✔ In the autumn, young ready-to-lay pullets are mixed in with the flock of older hens.

✔ Everything seems to be going well, until one to six weeks later, when many of the young pullets start sneezing, coughing, and looking droopy. They have thick, stinky snot coming out of their nostrils and eyes. Some of them have trouble breathing, and about one out of ten of the young birds die. The adult hens seem fine, but egg production drops in the flock.

To reduce the chances of your birds getting infectious coryza, you should bring home only day-old chicks from known sources. Don't mix different age groups; the older chickens will pass their infections on to this year's hatchlings and feed the vicious cycle.

A vaccine is available to protect chickens against infectious coryza, but it isn't commonly used in backyard flocks. Erythromycin, tetracycline, and sulfa drugs help affected birds survive and feel better quicker, but antibiotic treatment doesn't eliminate the disease from the flock. Some flock keepers embark on the long and expensive process of testing the flock and removing infected birds to eliminate the disease. Unfortunately, depopulation is the quickest, most effective method to eradicate it.

Mycoplasmosis

Mycoplasma gallisepticum, often just called MG, is the cause of chronic respiratory disease (CRD) of chickens. Coughing, noisy breathing, foamy eyes, and runny nostrils are typical signs of MG infection in backyard chickens, such as the one in Figure 12-1.

This disease is a chicken head cold that never goes away, or keeps coming back. For some reason, male birds tend to get bad cases of CRD, and the disease is more severe in cold weather.

The infection spreads rapidly in a flock after it's introduced, but many birds don't show any signs of it. Although MG is extremely common in backyard flocks, most flock owners never know it's there because the disease is so mild. Surveys suggest the chance that your flock is infected with MG (and you don't know it) is greater than 30 percent.

Bird-to-bird transmission is the most common way the germ gets around. Healthy-looking birds can carry MG lifelong and spread the infection. An infected hen can also pass MG to her chicks through the eggs, but this transmission happens at a low rate — maybe 3 to 5 percent of the eggs from an MG-infected hen will contain the bacteria.

Even with extreme biosecurity, keeping a flock MG-clean is challenging. Obtaining hatching eggs or day-old birds from MG-clean flocks is a great way to start, but for many popular backyard breeds, sources of MG-clean stock don't exist.

Antibiotic treatment doesn't eliminate the infection from a flock, but the birds usually feel better quicker with treatment. Erythromycin, tetracycline, and tylosin are among the antibiotics that usually work well to clear up signs of disease.

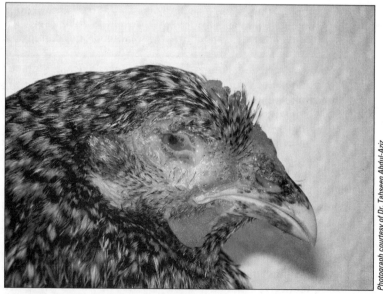

Photograph courtesy of Dr. Tahseen Abdul-Aziz

Figure 12-1: A chicken with mycoplasmosis.

Besides depopulation and starting over, other strategies have been used to clean up MG-infected flocks, including testing and removing MG-positive birds or treating hatching eggs with heat or antibiotic dips.

Necrotic enteritis

Necrotic enteritis (NE) is a disease of young chickens (2 weeks to 6 months) caused by infection with toxin-producing *Clostridium perfringens* bacteria. The disease also goes by the names *enterotoxemia* and *rot gut,* and it's a common problem of growing meat-type birds.

Diarrhea, severe depression, reluctance to move, and ruffled feathers are the signs seen in a flock during a necrotic enteritis outbreak. The disease can quickly kill birds.

The parasitic disease *coccidiosis* predisposes chickens to necrotic enteritis, so control of coccidia is important for NE prevention (see Chapter 13). Clean bedding and probiotics also reduce the chance of an outbreak. You can use bacitracin, lincomycin, tetracycline, or tylosin to treat sick birds.

Pullorum disease and fowl typhoid

Pullorum disease (PD) and *fowl typhoid (FT)* are two very similar poultry diseases; particular strains of *Salmonella* bacteria cause them both. (Scientists are still debating about the names of these strains, so we'll stay out of it.) In the United States, the National Poultry Improvement Program (NPIP), started in 1935, has nearly eliminated PD and FT from the country through testing and certifying pullorum-typhoid clean flocks.

Both diseases are transmitted bird-to-bird by carrier chickens. An infected hen passes them to her chicks through her eggs. Chicks hatched from PD- or FT-infected eggs die soon after hatching, between one day and one month. Affected chicks may gasp for air and have whitish diarrhea that causes pasty vents. Survivors are stunted. Fowl typhoid can affect older birds as well as chicks.

Get your chicks or hatching eggs from pullorum-typhoid clean flocks. Flock keepers in the United States can enroll their flocks in the NPIP program and have their birds tested by contacting their state veterinarian.

Treating Infectious Diseases Caused by Viruses

A *virus* is a tiny infectious agent that makes a living by hijacking a host and using the host's cells to reproduce. Viruses can't multiply outside of a living host, which can be an animal, plant, or bacteria, depending on the preference of the virus. In this section, we're only concerned about the viruses that have a taste for chicken.

Generally, antibiotics have no effect against viruses. The host must live long enough for the immune system to fight off the invader, so supportive care of the patient is the way to treat viral infections.

Avian encephalomyelitis

When a hen is infected by *avian encephalomyelitis (AE)* virus, she passes the virus to her chicks through her eggs for a short period of time only — about one week. After the infected chicks hatch, they spread the virus to their hatch mates. AE virus is so widespread that nearly all flocks of chickens eventually become infected with it.

The disease affects chicks from hatch day to several weeks of age, but most frequently between 1 and 3 weeks old. The main signs are unsteadiness, head and neck tremors, partial paralysis, or inability to move. The tremors from AE are more obvious if you hold an affected chick on its back in your cupped hands. Usually, about half of the chicks in a hatch will be affected, and somewhere between 25 to 60 percent will die from the infection. Although AE virus infects adult chickens, they show few signs of disease — only slightly decreased egg production in hens.

After AE virus enters a flock for the first time, natural immunity eventually develops. Hens raised in that flock pass protective antibodies in their eggs to their offspring, and outbreaks of AE in chicks eventually stop. In uninfected flocks, vaccination of hens against AE can provide immunity to their offspring.

No specific treatment is available for AE. With good nursing care, a few chicks recover completely. Survivors may develop cataracts in their eyes, resulting in blindness.

Avian influenza

Depending on the strain, *avian influenza (AI)* infections in poultry can range from no signs to severe illness and death of nearly

100 percent of the flock. Most strains of AI cause mild disease in chickens, but rare, deadly strains of AI cause droopy birds with sneezing, coughing, difficulty breathing, and runny eyes and nostrils. Comb and wattles may swell and turn purplish. You may also notice diarrhea and nervous system signs, such as a twisted neck.

Avian influenza is incredibly contagious and spreads rapidly in poultry flocks. In infected birds, the virus is present in the mucous coming from the eyes and nostrils, and in large amounts in the droppings. Contact with droppings and mucous are the main ways the infection is spread bird-to-bird. Dirty eggshells can be a source of infection for chicks in an incubator.

 Good biosecurity practices are important to prevent introducing AI to backyard flocks. Don't share equipment with other flock keepers, unless it has been cleaned and disinfected. Quarantine new birds for 30 days before letting them meet your flock. Refer to Chapter 4 for biosecurity measures you can take.

 Report the sudden deaths of a large number of birds to your state veterinarian or other animal health official, because these sudden deaths can be a sign of a deadly, highly contagious strain of avian influenza. Animal health officials want to act quickly to stop an outbreak from becoming widespread.

Chicken infectious anemia

The *chicken infectious anemia (CIA)* virus causes 2- to 3-week-old chicks to become listless and pale. Death occurs in less than 30 percent of cases, usually because the virus depresses the chick's immune system, allowing bacteria to invade. Surviving chicks recover in a few weeks.

Chickens of all ages can become infected with CIA virus, but only young chicks show problems. The virus is spread bird to bird through body fluids and droppings. Recently infected hens pass the virus in their eggs, and roosters can spread it through semen.

 Vaccinating hens can prevent CIA disease in their chicks, because the hens pass antibodies in their eggs. Hens that were infected with CIA virus as youngsters also give protective antibodies to their offspring. No specific treatment is available for CIA, but antibiotics can reduce chick deaths due to secondary bacterial infections.

Fowl pox

Fowl pox is a long, drawn-out viral infection in chicken and turkey flocks. The disease has two forms:

✔ **Dry form:** This form of fowl pox causes crusty scabs and wart-like lumps on the comb, wattles, eyelids, and other featherless areas of skin. The dry form is the milder and more common version of the disease.

✔ **Wet form:** This form of fowl pox affects the inside of the bird, making sores in the mouth, throat, and windpipe. These birds obviously feel very ill. Up to 50 percent of the flock may die, either from suffocation or because they're unable to eat or drink.

In an individual bird, fowl pox usually runs its course in about two weeks, but flock outbreaks can drag out for two to three months. An affected flock grows poorly, and egg production drops.

The virus enters a bird's body through a scratch or other wound in the skin, or through the mucous membranes of the eye and mouth. Infected birds or insects, especially mosquitoes, which carry the virus from one place to another, can introduce fowl pox to a flock. Scabs fall off affected birds and contaminate the flock's environment with fowl pox virus, which can remain infectious in the soil for many months.

You can prevent fowl pox from entering your flock with good biosecurity practices, including quarantining new birds, keeping your birds at home, and controlling biting insects. Fowl pox vaccine is available and practical for backyard flock keepers to give, so consider vaccinating if you live in an area where fowl pox is rampant.

After fowl pox enters a flock, vaccination is a helpful tool to control outbreaks. You can administer the vaccine to your chickens in the skin of the wing web, using a simple tool. The vaccine contains live virus that stimulates the bird's immune system by producing a mild form of the disease. Chicks can be vaccinated starting at one day old. In regions where mosquitoes are active year-round, vaccinating twice a year is a good idea.

Good nursing care helps chickens survive fowl pox. Following are a few more suggestions for supportive care:

✔ **Give antibiotics in drinking water to control secondary bacterial infections.** Tetracycline is your best choice for this purpose.

✔ **Swab the scabby areas of skin with a dilute iodine solution to speed healing.** You can later apply a fly repellent ointment to soften scabs and keep irritating and disease-spreading mosquitoes away. We provide a homemade recipe for a fly repellent ointment in the appendix.

> ✔ **Mix diluted iodine solutions into the flock's drinking water.**
> Doing so seems to reduce deaths due to the severe, wet form
> of the disease; see the appendix for the recipe.

Infectious bronchitis

The *infectious bronchitis (IB)* virus causes respiratory disease,
mostly in young chickens, and infects the reproductive tract of
hens. Here are the signs:

✔ **Young chickens:** They experience gasping, coughing, sneezing, and runny eyes and nostrils. In general, younger chicks
have more severe signs. You may not notice the infection in
older chicks unless you visit the coop at night when the flock
is resting and listen for sneezing (sneezing chickens make a
distinctive "snicking" sound).

✔ **Hens:** They have decreased egg production with ugly eggs.
The insides as well as the outsides of the eggs are abnormal;
egg whites are watery; and egg shells are thin, rough, or wrin-
kly. Egg production improves after six to eight weeks, but it
usually doesn't return to the level it was before IB infection.
Hens may or may not have mild respiratory signs.

IB is very contagious and spreads fast in a flock. Infected chickens
can shed the virus off and on for months in snot and droppings,
contaminating everything in the flock's living space. People can
spread the infection with dirty shoes, hands, and equipment.
Prevention of IB is another good reason for biosecurity. Use an
all-in, all-out system for your flock if possible (see Chapter 4), and
bring home only day-old chicks from known sources.

Vaccination controls IB on multi-age chicken farms to prevent ugly
eggs and poor egg production. No specific treatment is available
for IB, but keeping the brooder area slightly warmer seems to help
chicks recover, and antibiotics may ward off secondary bacterial
infections.

Infectious bursal disease

Infectious bursal disease (IBD), sometimes called *Gumboro* after the
town of Gumboro, Delaware, where IBD was first discovered, is a
highly contagious disease of young birds. The disease is a major
problem for meat-type birds on commercial farms, but so far it
hasn't caused much grief for backyard flocks.

IBD has two basic forms, depending on the age of the chick and the strain of the IBD virus:

- ✔ **Younger chick:** If chicks are infected with the IBD virus at an early age, before 3 weeks old, they don't show outward signs of disease but their immune systems are severely and permanently damaged. They don't grow well, and they often die of other infections a short time later.

- ✔ **Older chick:** Chicks between 3 and 6 weeks old suddenly get sick from IBD infection. They're droopy and tremble or stagger. They have diarrhea, pasty butts, and peck at each other's vents. Nearly all the birds in the group will be affected in the course of a week or two, and up to 20 percent may die. The immune system damage is temporary, in this case.

Infected chickens shed the virus in their poop, contaminating feed, water, and bedding. Other chickens pick up the virus by ingesting that stuff. The virus is fairly hardy outside of a chicken's body, so people can spread it on shoes, hands, and equipment. The best way you can prevent IBD is to use good biosecurity practices that we discuss in Chapter 4.

Vaccination controls the disease on commercial poultry farms. Because of cost, lack of availability, and tricky timing of booster shots, the IBD vaccination is rarely used in backyard flocks. No specific treatment is available for IBD, only good nursing care.

Infectious laryngotracheitis

Infectious laryngotracheitis (ILT) is a viral respiratory infection of adult chickens, and this one is nasty. Affected chickens gasp for air and sling bloody mucous from their open mouths, staining their feathers and those of flock mates. It's no surprise that flock egg production decreases precipitously.

The disease runs its course in about two weeks. Some strains of the virus don't kill many birds, but the mortality rate from bad strains may be as high as 50 percent of the flock. Cause of death is often suffocation due to blood clots in the windpipe.

After chickens have recovered from ILT, they can carry the virus for life and shed it during stressful times. These carrier chickens are the main source of infection for other flocks. The virus doesn't last long in the environment, so contaminated poultry equipment and people's dirty hands and shoes are less important in spreading the infection than carrier birds. The moral of the story is: Don't bring adult chickens home to meet your flock.

Widespread ILT outbreaks have happened just after major poultry shows, when birds from several regions mixed in the show hall and then returned home with a virus souvenir. If you show poultry, consider vaccinating your flock for ILT to protect your valuable breeding stock. See Chapter 16 for more information on ILT vaccine.

No specific treatment is available for ILT, except to make it as easy as possible for birds to breathe. You can provide a relatively dust-free environment and avoid disturbing the flock. Vaccinating healthy birds in the early stages of a flock outbreak may limit losses.

Lymphoid leukosis

Lymphoid leukosis is a disease of adult chickens caused by *avian leukosis virus (ALV)*. This virus causes tumors to develop in the internal organs of a small proportion of infected chickens. Because the liver is the common site of those tumors, lymphoid leukosis is also known as "big liver disease." Although ALV is everywhere — most flocks are probably infected — lymphoid leukosis affects only a few members of the flock, maybe 1 to 2 percent.

Backyard flock keepers may not recognize lymphoid leukosis as the cause of death for a single hen who seemed to just fade away, unless a postmortem is performed to discover the tumors.

Outward signs of lymphoid leukosis are usually vague and not very specific. They include loss of appetite, weakness, diarrhea, and wasting. You may sometimes notice more specific signs, such as an enlarged abdomen, swollen legs, shriveled comb, or bleeding from spots where feathers enter the skin. Affected chickens die within a few weeks.

An infected hen transmits the virus to her chicks through her eggs. When these infected chicks hatch, they spread the virus to hatch mates. Chickens that develop tumors are usually the ones that got their infection from their mothers, rather than from hatch mates.

Unfortunately, you can't do much about this disease; it has no vaccination or treatment. Commercial poultry companies have managed to eradicate ALV from elite breeding stock by testing and using only ALV-free parents and by hatching chicks in small groups.

Marek's disease

Marek's disease (MD) virus is so common, everywhere in the world, that you have to assume that your flock has been exposed to the virus, whether your birds show signs or not. Although the virus is highly contagious and nearly every bird in the flock may become infected, only a small proportion of birds infected with the MD virus actually develop the disease.

Marek's disease virus is another tumor-causing virus, like ALV. Marek's disease, however, can affect chickens as young as 1 month old, whereas lymphoid leukosis doesn't show up until birds are at least 4 months old.

The virus is easily transmitted from chicken to chicken, especially through feather dander and dust, on which the virus can live for many months. MD isn't egg transmitted. The four forms of MD are as follows:

- ✓ **Skin form:** A chicken has red, enlarged feather follicles or white bumps on the skin with brown, crusty scabs. MD affects feathered skin, which is different from fowl pox, which causes scabs on featherless areas of skin.

- ✓ **Nerve form:** A chicken suffers paralysis of a wing or a leg with this form. One leg held forward and one leg held backward is a classic sign of MD. You can see this split-leg pose in Figure 12-2. Birds may also have diarrhea or difficulty breathing or develop a crop impaction.

- ✓ **Eye form:** The colored iris of one or both eyes turns gray, and the pupil is misshapen, not round like it should be. The bird becomes blind in the affected eye or eyes.

- ✓ **Internal organ form:** Tumors develop in the internal organs, causing a variety of signs, depending on the tumor location. Affected birds don't eat; they lose weight and look droopy. You may notice an enlarged abdomen or mistakenly think that a hen with an abdominal tumor is egg-bound.

Marek's disease is nearly always fatal. Some birds with the nerve form of the disease may appear to get better after a few days, but often they die a short time later from their tumors. With little hope for recovery and no treatment for MD, euthanasia is the most humane option for suffering birds.

Marek's disease vaccination doesn't protect against infection with the virus, but it does a good job of preventing tumors and death from the disease. To be effective, the vaccine must be given as early as possible in a chick's life. If you order day-old chicks from a mail-order hatchery that offers chick MD vaccination, say yes!

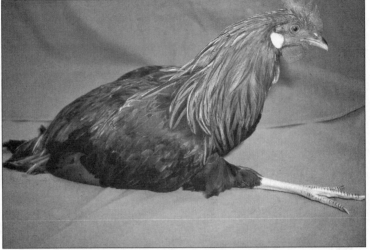

Photograph courtesy of Dr. Tahseen Abdul-Aziz

Figure 12-2: Split-leg pose of a chicken with Marek's disease.

Many commercial poultry producers now vaccinate chicks in the egg before they're hatched, using automated equipment and cutting-edge vaccine. Backyard flock keepers have access to a lower-tech vaccine that is given to day-old chicks; this old vaccine may still be helpful, and we recommend it.

All's not lost if vaccination isn't feasible for you. Chicks become more resistant to infection with MD virus as they grow up. Knowing that, you can take steps to protect your chicks from MD:

- ✔ Isolate your chicks from other chickens until they are 5 months old.

- ✔ Choose an isolation area that hasn't been used to house older birds for long time. Thoroughly clean and disinfect the place to remove dust and dander, before putting chicks in it.

Newcastle disease

The strain of this disease really makes a difference in how severe your flock is affected. Newcastle disease virus strains range in potency from no-big-deal to chicken Armageddon. Although many other types of birds, including poultry and pet birds, can be infected with and spread Newcastle disease virus, chickens tend to suffer most from the disease.

- ✔ **The mild form:** This form of Newcastle disease looks like a cold with a little sneezing and coughing. Egg production decreases and eggs are ugly, with watery whites and thin, splotchy, rough, or wrinkled eggshells. Mild strains of Newcastle disease virus are common wherever chickens are raised, including the United States.

✔ **The virulent form:** This form of Newcastle disease, called *exotic Newcastle disease* in the United States, severely affects the chicken's respiratory, digestive, and nervous systems. In addition to the respiratory signs and egg production problems, chickens may have swollen heads and watery, greenish diarrhea. Nervous system signs include twisted neck, walking in circles, tremors, droopy wings, and paralysis. Sudden death may be the only indication. The mortality rate can approach 100 percent of the flock in just a few days. Virulent strains aren't present in the United States at this time, and we want to keep it that way.

You can protect your hens against the negative egg production effects of mild forms of Newcastle disease by vaccinating them as pullets.

Like avian influenza, exotic strains of Newcastle disease are highly contagious and extremely deadly for chickens. Report the sudden deaths of a large number of birds to your state veterinarian or other animal health official, who will want to act quickly to stop an outbreak from becoming widespread.

Chapter 13

Exterminating Chicken Parasites and Other Creepy-Crawlies

. . . .

In This Chapter
▶ Recognizing common internal parasites, such as coccidia and worms
▶ Identifying what's pestering you and your chickens: External parasites

. . . .

*B*ackyard chickens live in a wormy world, and they're also plagued by mites, lice, and other pests. All flocks have microscopic, single-celled coccidia parasites to some extent, and scientists estimate that more than 80 percent of backyard flocks play host to parasitic worms. In this chapter, we describe the main backyard flock creepy-crawlies, both internal and external, and what you can do about them.

Taking a Look Inside: Internal Parasites

The critters that affect your flock inside are especially bothersome. In fact, several decades ago farmers moved their birds inside to avoid parasitic worms. Now that free-range and backyard poultry flock keepers are putting chickens back outside, parasitic worms are enjoying a comeback. In these sections, we give you some suggestions on how you can handle intestinal parasite problems.

Coccidiosis

Coccidiosis is such a common and serious problem for flock keepers everywhere. Microscopic coccidia parasites are the archenemies of poultry farmers, who must spend tremendous amounts of effort and money to keep coccidiosis at bay. The parasites can multiply to overwhelming numbers in the digestive tracts of chickens, usually young ones, causing bloody or watery diarrhea, poor growth, and death.

Every chicken carries a few coccidia around. You can see what the eggs, or *oocysts*, look like at the microscopic level in a sample of the droppings (flip ahead to Figure 13-2). What makes the difference between healthy chickens with a few coccidia and a flock that's really sick with coccidiosis? Check out these factors:

✔ **The number of oocysts eaten:** Chickens raised in crowded or unsanitary conditions are exposed to heavy doses of oocysts every day.

✔ **The strain of coccidia:** Some strains are more vicious than others and burrow deeper into the gut.

✔ **The environment:** Coccidia like warm, wet conditions. Freezing weather and drought conditions kill oocysts.

✔ **The chicken's age and health status:** Chickens develop immunity to coccidia as they grow older. Young chickens between 3 to 5 weeks of age are most susceptible. Chickens that are run down by other diseases or poor nutrition are also more susceptible to coccidiosis.

Preventing coccidiosis

Besides taking no action and hoping for the best, you have these two choices for preventing a coccidiosis outbreak in your young chickens (you can do one or the other, but not both):

✔ **Use a medicated starter feed for chicks until they're 4 months old.** The anticoccidial medication in the feed doesn't kill all the oocysts, but it keeps them down to a dull roar while chicks develop immunity.

✔ **Have your day-old chicks vaccinated with a coccidiosis vaccine.** Some hatcheries offer this service, or you may be able to purchase the vaccine and do it yourself. The vaccine is actually a live, mild strain of coccidia that stimulates chicks' immunity to natural infection with more aggressive versions of coccidia. After vaccinating chicks, *don't* feed medicated feed; doing so defeats the purpose of the vaccine.

Here are important steps to controlling coccidiosis, regardless of whether you medicate, vaccinate, or neither:

✔ **Keep pens clean and dry, and avoid overcrowding.** Keep poop out of feeders and waterers. Coccidia love wet conditions, especially sloppy areas around waterers. Remove wet bedding frequently and replace with dry stuff.

The attack and spread of the coccidia

So how exactly do coccidia infect your chickens and make them sick? The life story of a coccidial organism starts when the egg stage (called an *oocyst*) is shed from the lining of a chicken's intestine and passes in the bird's droppings. On the ground, the oocyst matures for a couple of days into a *sporulated oocyst,* a form of the parasite that is capable of infecting another chicken, and then it patiently waits to be eaten. (Depending on conditions, oocysts can wait many months.)

After another chicken unknowingly eats the oocyst while scratching and pecking on the ground, the parasite travels to the intestine or the ceca and burrows in. There, inside the cells of the gut, the organism gets busy, dividing many times and destroying many intestinal cells in the process. Eventually, thousands of the oocyst's offspring are shed in the droppings, to continue the cycle.

✔ **Raise chicks on wire-floored brooders.** You may need to take this step if the flock has had coccidiosis problems in past years and the environment has become heavily contaminated with oocysts.

✔ **Treat birds with signs of coccidiosis immediately.** Amprolium or sulfa drugs beat back coccidiosis. Check out the appendix for more information about coccidiosis treatments.

How do you know if chickens are suffering from coccidiosis? Chicks are pale and droopy, with ruffled feathers and no appetite. They pass bloody or watery diarrhea. You notice the greatest amount of blood in the droppings four or five days after the signs start, which is also when most deaths occur. You may see the poor birds walk back and forth to the feeder, crying pitifully, but not eating. Chicks that survive longer than a week are on the road to recovery.

Treatment of coccidiosis

Amprolium or sulfa drugs effectively treat coccidiosis outbreaks. The parasites can develop resistance to these drugs, but so far, resistance isn't a common problem in backyard flocks. Organic poultry farmers have a tough time controlling coccidiosis, but they have used vinegar in the drinking water or the dried leaves of the wormwood plant in the feed with some success.

Be careful though when administering sulfa drugs. Your birds can easily overdose on it, causing toxic effects, so take care to mix sulfa drug solutions according to label directions.

Parasitic worms

A zoo of parasitic worms can be found in chicken flocks. Worms find cozy places to stay in the crop, gizzard, intestine, cecum, windpipe, and even the eyelids.

Figure 13-1 displays the mug shots of the most common chicken worms. We discuss these worms in greater depth in these sections.

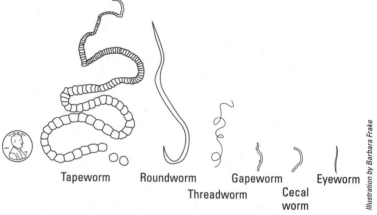

Tapeworm   Roundworm   Gapeworm   Eyeworm
Threadworm   Cecal worm

Illustration by Barbara Frake

Figure 13-1: A wide array of parasitic worms in chickens compared to the size of a penny.

The eggs and immature stages of many parasitic worms can live outside of the chicken host for a long time, possibly several years. Some parasitic worms spend part of their lifecycle in other creatures, such as earthworms, insects, slugs, or snails. Chickens pick up worms by eating dirt or litter contaminated with worm eggs or by eating small creatures carrying immature stages of worms.

Cecal worm

Cecal worms, also called *heterakis worms,* reside in the ceca of chickens. They're very common and generally don't do much harm. The main worry with cecal worms is their ability to carry blackhead parasites, which are deadly for turkeys but rarely cause disease in chickens.

Eyeworm

Eyeworms *(Oxyspirura mansoni)* cause trouble only in warm climates, such as the southeastern United States, where the particular cockroach host lives. The parasite burrows under the third eyelid of chickens and other birds, causing eye to swell shut.

As you can imagine, it's irritating, and the bird does additional damage by scratching at the eye.

Gapeworm

Syngamus trachea, the gapeworm, attaches to the lining of the windpipe in chickens and other poultry. If enough gapeworms get together in the windpipe, they cause a disease known as *the gapes,* named for the open-mouthed, distressed breathing of affected chickens. Young birds are more likely than older birds to have heavy infestations of gapeworms and get the gapes, which can be fatal.

Roundworm

Roundworms *(Ascaridia galli)* are by far the most common parasitic worm of chickens. Young chickens with heavy infections of these big intestinal worms get skinny despite a good appetite. Chickens older than 4 months develop resistance to roundworms; the mature chicken's immune system kicks out most of the bums.

Every once in a while a roundworm will crawl into a hen's oviduct and wind up inside an egg that she lays. This isn't a human health hazard; it's just disgusting.

Tapeworm

Long ribbon-shaped tapeworms live in chickens' intestines, where they don't eat much or (usually) do much damage. In large numbers, tapeworms can cause birds to be skinny, but they're rarely fatal.

Threadworm

Some *Capillaria,* or threadworms, hang out in the crop or esophagus; others prefer to live in the intestinal lining. Heavy infections cause droopiness, pale combs, weight loss, and sometimes death.

Diagnosing parasitic worm infections

A veterinary diagnostic laboratory or veterinarian's office can diagnose intestinal worm infections by examining droppings under a microscope for parasite eggs or by postmortem. Small animal veterinarians may not be very familiar with chicken parasites, and some flock keepers armed with a microscope may want to take a look themselves, so we include drawings of chicken intestinal parasites in Figure 13-2 to show you what they look like.

Treating and preventing parasitic worms

You can't completely eradicate parasitic worms, so the goal is to knock down their numbers by deworming so they do no harm to their hosts. To *deworm* your chickens means you give a medication that is effective at killing or paralyzing intestinal worms. The dead or dying worms pass out of the chicken's intestines in the droppings.

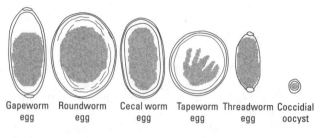

Gapeworm egg   Roundworm egg   Cecal worm egg   Tapeworm egg   Threadworm egg   Coccidial oocyst

Illustration by Barbara Frake

Figure 13-2: Chicken intestinal parasites under the microscope.

Be careful about deworming too much. Repeated deworming only leads to worms developing resistance to medications. Good evidence actually suggests that hosting a few worms is an immune system booster, believe it or not!

Albendazole, fenbendazole, ivermectin, and levamisole are effective treatments for most parasitic worms of chickens. Fenbendazole and albendazole have the advantage of being extremely safe medications. Piperazine is only effective against roundworms. See the appendix for dosages.

In the United States, legal use of any dewormer medications for chickens (except for piperazine in non-laying chickens) requires a prescription from a veterinarian. Talk to your veterinarian about timing of treatment and egg discard times.

We're still waiting for an effective herbal or mineral remedy for chicken worms. Tobacco is far too toxic. We had high hopes for diatomaceous earth (DE), but extensive research has had very disappointing results; the substance has little if any effect against internal parasites. (If you're a DE fan, read on. The stuff can be used to fight external parasites — lice and mites.) The dried leaves of *Artemisia* herbs (wormwood and sweet Annie) seem promising, so we're keeping our eyes on those and other herbal dewormer studies.

Completely keeping your chickens away from worms isn't possible. Even if it were, we don't advise it. With good management on your part, worms may never cause illness in your flock. Good nutrition and a clean environment are very important in preventing heavy worm infections and illness due to parasites. Here are other things that flock keepers who don't have a parasite problem usually do well:

✔ **Manage chickens:**

- **Give the birds plenty of room.** Avoid overcrowding.
- **Try not to introduce wormy chickens to the flock.** Get your chicks as day-olds or deworm older birds before letting them meet your flock.

- **Remove (cull) birds with repeated parasite problems.** Some animals are just inclined to being wormy (it may be a genetic predisposition). Those few chronically wormy individuals are responsible for most of the worm burden in the flock and most of the contamination of the environment with worm eggs.

✔ **Manage the flock's environment:**

- **Rotate and rest pastures for pastured poultry.** Periodically move the chickens to different ground, and leave the old site empty of birds for several months or years, if possible.

- **Keep wild birds away from the flock.** They may be infected and shedding worm eggs in their droppings.

- **Keep chickens off freshly tilled ground.** Doing so greatly reduces the amount of feasting on the banquet of turned-up earthworms and insects.

- **Use integrated pest management (IPM) practices to control insect populations.** Integrated pest management is an environmentally sensitive approach to pest management that relies on a combination of common-sense practices, such as rotating pastures and using mechanical trapping devices before resorting to broad-spectrum chemical pesticides. For more about using IPM for your flock in the United States, contact your local extension office.

Other internal parasites

Besides coccidiosis and parasitic worms, a few other parasites occasionally cause problems for backyard flocks, and they deserve honorable mention here.

Blackhead (Histomoniasis)

Carried by cecal worms and earthworms, the organisms that cause blackhead are parasites within parasites. Blackhead is a serious problem for turkeys but not so much for chickens, who usually get a mild "droopy bird" illness. Controlling cecal worms with dewormers controls blackhead.

Canker (Trichomoniasis)

Canker is primarily a disease of pigeons and doves, but chickens can get it, too. The trichomonad parasites invade a bird's mouth, sinuses, esophagus, and crop, causing yellowish fluffy growths. Canker can be spread by close contact between birds and by contaminated water. An avian veterinarian can diagnose the condition and provide treatment options.

Cryptosporidiosis

Cryptosporidiosis mostly causes respiratory disease in meat-type chickens under 3 weeks old, especially chicks that have damaged immune systems due to infectious bursal disease. No treatment exists for cryptosporidiosis.

Toxoplasmosis

Toxoplasmosis is a disease of free-range flocks that are exposed to cat poop or have the opportunity to eat dead rodents. This is the same disease that causes illness in people, cats, and other animals. In chickens, toxoplasmosis causes weight loss, blindness, and problems with the nervous system. This disease is yet another reason why cats, rats, and mice don't belong in chicken pens.

Examining the Outside: External Parasites

Poultry lice and mites are extremely common external parasites of chickens. You can spot these critters before they get out of control if you periodically pick up and examine chickens in your flock. Figure 13-3 gives you an up-close look at poultry lice and mites that you may see during your routine bug check. The following sections explain these critters in greater detail.

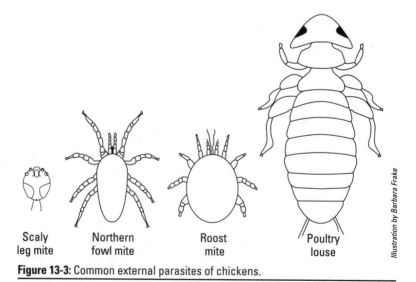

Scaly leg mite | Northern fowl mite | Roost mite | Poultry louse

Illustration by Barbara Frake

Figure 13-3: Common external parasites of chickens.

Poultry lice

Poultry lice are wingless, straw-colored insects that feed on dry skin scales, scabs, and feathers. A poultry louse spends its entire life on its bird host; if it falls off the bird, it won't survive long in the environment — maybe a few days. Lice know what they like, and poultry lice like chickens, not people or pets. If a poultry louse climbs on you, it won't stay long.

Louse infestations are a drag, especially for young chickens, making them jumpy and slow to grow. Fertility and egg production declines for infested adults. The plumage of lousy birds looks patchy and moth-eaten.

Female lice lay their eggs *(nits)* in clumps on feather shafts (see Figure 13-4). Inspect birds at least twice a month, spreading the feathers in the vent, breast, and thigh areas, looking for nit clumps or pale, scurrying insects. Fall and winter are when most louse infestations are common.

A menu of mites

Mites are tiny relatives of ticks and spiders. A long list of mites infest chickens, so we just concentrate on three of the most common types of chicken-loving mites in these sections.

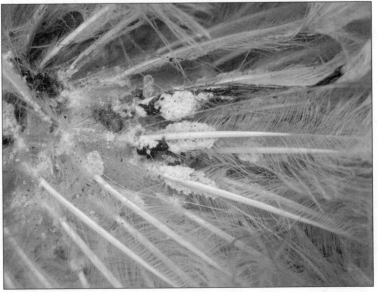

Photograph courtesy of Dr. Tahseen Abdul-Aziz

Figure 13-4: Louse eggs on feather shafts.

Northern fowl mite

The *northern fowl mite* is a serious pest of poultry, and this mite has also been found scurrying on wild birds, rats, and people. These mites are blood-suckers, and in heavy infestations, they can cause blood loss, stunted growth, decreased egg production, weakness, and even death. They eat anytime, day or night.

The mites congregate in the vent area; feathers there may be blackened by mites and mite excrement (we show an example in Figure 13-5). If you pick up and handle a bird with northern fowl mites, the mites climbing your arms and hands may creep you out.

Four main sources can introduce the northern fowl mite to your flock:

✓ Chickens

✓ Transport coops

✓ People

✓ Wild birds

To patrol for a northern fowl mite infestation in your flock, pick up and examine the vent areas of several birds every two weeks.

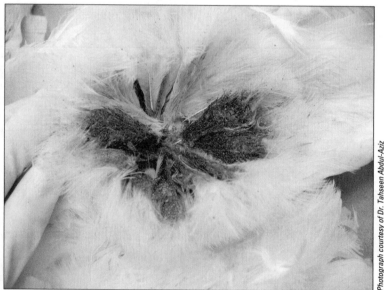

Photograph courtesy of Dr. Tahseen Abdul-Aziz

Figure 13-5: Northern fowl mites infesting a hen's vent area.

Roost mite

The *roost mite,* also known as the *red mite* or *chicken mite,* is also a blood-sucker that feeds on poultry and wild birds. The roost mite has a different modus operandi, however; it feeds on chickens only at night and hides in the coop, on roosts, or under piles of droppings during the day.

 To spot a roost mite infestation, you need to examine birds at night, looking for dark moving specks, or inspect the coop. Roost mites congregate in cracks and crevices inside chicken houses, seen as tiny red or blackish dots clustered together. Another tip-off: Hens may refuse to lay in infested nests.

Roost mites are spread the same way as northern fowl mites (see the preceding section): poultry, people, equipment, and wild birds (pigeons, especially). They're difficult to eradicate from poultry premises, even after the chickens are gone, because roost mites can live for months without eating.

Scaly leg mite

Scaly leg mites spend their entire lives in the skin of their bird hosts, burrowing tunnels under the scales of the legs and sometimes into the skin of the combs and wattles. Crusty scabs and lumps appear on the scales of the legs of older birds (check out Figure 13-6). Long-term infestations result in deformed toes and limping. Scaly leg mites are transmitted bird to bird and by contact with an infested bird's environment.

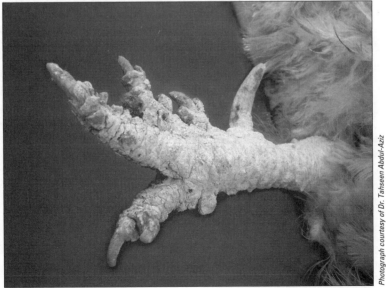

Photograph courtesy of Dr. Tahseen Abdul-Aziz

Figure 13-6: The effects of scaly leg mites.

Scaly leg mites are too small to be seen without a microscope. If you suspect a scaly leg mite infestation, you can scrape crusts from an affected bird's leg, put the scrapings in a container, and have a veterinarian or diagnostic laboratory examine the sample.

Preventing and treating lice and mites

Lice and mites are born slobs; they like a damp and dirty coop, so general cleanliness can make your coop less hospitable to these unwelcome guests. Here are some additional measures to protect your flock:

- ✓ **Quarantine all new birds for 30 days before letting them meet your flock.** Inspect new birds for external parasites at least twice during the quarantine period and treat them if necessary. See Chapter 4 for more explanation.

- ✓ **Thoroughly clean transport coops after use.** You can dislodge hitchhiking pests with a thorough cleaning.

- ✓ **Discourage wild birds from hanging out with your flock.** To do so, use bird netting, screened coop windows, or scare tactics.

To control lice or mites, you can treat both the birds and the birds' environment. Because roost mites spend so much time off the chicken and living in the coop, treating only the birds will fail to eliminate the problem. If you diagnose poultry lice, northern fowl mite, or roost mites, treat all the birds in the flock at the same time. Isolate any chickens with scaly leg mite from the rest of the flock while they're being treated.

Be patient, and don't expect to get the situation under control with one shot; repeated treatments are necessary. Lice and mites can develop resistance to pesticides, so vary your method and alternate treatments. In Table 13-1, we list some methods that you can safely use to control external parasites. You can find more information about these treatments in the appendix.

Table 13-1   External Parasite Treatments for Chickens

Pesticide	Effective against	Uses	Forms
Camphor	Scaly leg mite	Chicken's legs and feet	Ointment
Diatomaceous earth (DE)	Lice, northern fowl mite, roost mite	Chicken, coop, dustbath	Powder
Garlic juice	Northern fowl mite	Chicken	Spray
Ivermectin	Lice, northern fowl mite, roost mite, scaly leg mite	Chicken	By mouth or injection, prescribed by a veterinarian
Neem oil	Lice, northern fowl mite, roost mite	Chicken, coop	Spray
Petroleum jelly/sulfur mix	Scaly leg mite	Chicken's legs and feet	Ointment
Pyrethrin and permethrin	Lice, northern fowl mite, roost mite	Chicken, coop	Powder, spray, dip
Sulfur	Lice, northern fowl mite, roost mite	Chicken, coop, dustbath	Powder, spray

 An easy way to dust birds with a powder-form pesticide (such as permethrin, DE, or sulfur) is to place the powder and the chicken in a garbage bag (leaving the chicken's head out of the bag!). Hold the bag closed around the chicken's neck, and shake the bag to distribute the powder all over the chicken's body.

 Or, even easier, let the chickens dust themselves. Build a dust-bath box (24 x 24 x 8 inches is a nice size) and fill it with a mix of playground sand and either diatomaceous earth (50:50 sand: DE) or sulfur powder (75:25 sand: sulfur). Sulfur powder, available at garden stores, has especially good residual action against mites and lice.

Chiggers, fleas, and bedbugs: Are you itching yet?

Have you seen chiggers, fleas, and bedbugs? Take a look at a lineup of a few other suspects in Figure 13-7. These are part-time pests, jumping on chickens for a meal and then bailing off. They may be a problem where you live. These bugs aren't fussy — they'll pester you as well as your chickens.

Bedbugs

Yes, this is the same *bedbug* that lives in people's homes and attacks them. They can move into a coop just as happily, hiding in crevices and taking blood meals from chickens. Unless you're okay with torching the coop and starting fresh, the best bet is to talk to an exterminator to get rid of them.

Chiggers

Chiggers mainly affect free-range chickens living in the southern United States. These mites live on the ground, preferring fence rows and brushy areas. Chiggers hunt in packs, clustering on chickens' wings, neck, and breast, and creating blisters where they attach and feed on the skin. Chigger attacks can be serious for small chicks. If you live where chiggers are a problem, pyrethrin sprays or sulfur dustbaths may repel these pests.

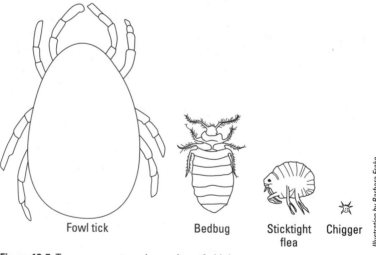

Fowl tick   Bedbug   Sticktight   Chigger
                                       flea

Illustration by Barbara Frake

Figure 13-7: Temporary external parasites of chickens.

Fowl ticks

Fowl ticks, or *blue bugs,* also like warmer climates. They feed on a variety of birds and occasionally mammals. The fowl tick's lifestyle is similar to that of the roost mite or bedbug; it lives in cracks and crevices of the coop and comes out to suck blood from chickens at night. Chickens heavily infested with fowl ticks can become weak and die. Thorough cleaning and spraying the coop with permethrin are appropriate control measures.

Sticktight fleas

Sticktight fleas cluster in large numbers around a chicken's eyes and on the wattles. The fleas embed their mouthparts deep in the sensitive skin, taking a meal of blood and creating a lot of irritation. Blood loss can be serious for young chickens. To fight back, we suggest using permethrin dust or smothering the fleas with petroleum jelly.

Chapter 14

Identifying Miscellaneous and Mystery Chicken Diseases

● ●

In This Chapter

▶ Venturing into a fungal jungle of chicken health problems

▶ Managing fast-growing broilers to prevent breakdowns

▶ Dodging or patiently treating bumblefoot

▶ Diagnosing causes of the bulge on your chicken's neck

● ●

*N*ot every disease your chicken may come down with falls into the clear-cut categories of flock-management accidents, bacterial, viral, or parasitic diseases that we talk about in Chapters 11, 12, and 13. This odd collection of chicken diseases doesn't fit anywhere else, but they're important enough for backyard chickens that we need to talk about them. In this chapter, we describe three chicken infections caused by molds and yeasts, and we discuss some common problems that don't have a clear cause; multiple or mysterious factors are involved. Among these multifactorial diseases, bumblefoot and crop problems are issues that many flock keepers will eventually encounter. In each of the two sections, the diseases are listed in alphabetical order for easy reference.

Like the chapters about flock management accidents and bacterial, viral, and parasitic diseases, we don't mean to scare you with all the things that can go wrong. We just want to give you more information if you receive a specific diagnosis for your flock or if your chicken health advisor mentions a particular chicken ailment as a possibility.

Recognizing Fungal Infections: Molds and Yeasts

Sometimes your flock may come down with ailments caused by fungal infections. Fungi aren't plants or animals; they're a unique, primitive category of life all their own. Mushrooms, molds, and yeast are fungi. In this section, we're concerned with molds and yeasts, because they can infect and sicken backyard chickens under the right circumstances.

Brooder pneumonia (Aspergillosis)

Aspergillus mold organisms grow in every chicken's environment, flourishing in damp bedding and rotten coop wood. Healthy adult chickens aren't particularly bothered by a little mold, but when the environment is teeming with mold spores, young chicks or stressed, rundown adult birds can be overwhelmed.

Aspergillus causes different forms of aspergillosis. The most common form of *Aspergillus* mold infection is *brooder pneumonia,* a lung and air-sac disease of chicks. Less-common forms of aspergillosis affect eyes, skin, brain, or bones. Chicks affected by brooder pneumonia gasp, lose their appetite, and look sleepy. The disease doesn't spread from chick to chick, but the mold can infect many chicks in a group at once, and up to half may die from the infection.

Unfortunately no effective drug treatment or vaccination is available for brooder pneumonia. Good nursing care and eliminating mold from the environment helps chicks survive. You can prevent outbreaks of brooder pneumonia with these suggestions:

- **Start your chicks off right with a clean and disinfected brooder box or area.** Check for rotten wood or moldy spots on the floor and walls of the building where you brood your chicks. Remove rotting wood or treat any moldy spots with a fungicidal disinfectant before moving chicks in.

- **Use clean feed, hay, or straw.** Make sure none of them have any mold, which can lead to brooder pneumonia.

- **Clean chick feeders and waterers daily.** You can sanitize drinking water with household bleach (see the appendix). Remove wet bedding promptly and replace it with fresh, dry stuff.

Candidiasis (Thrush)

Candidiasis, also known as *thrush*, is caused by the yeast *Candida albicans*, and it affects the mouth, crop, gizzard, or vent of many types of birds, including chickens. Whitish, thickened patches form inside the crop or on the skin of the vent area of a chicken suffering from candidiasis. In a few cases, sores may develop in the gizzard's lining.

The outward signs of candidiasis aren't very obvious: Affected birds are thin, listless, and disheveled — they just don't feel very good. The yeast organism takes advantage of young, old, and sick birds, and isn't usually a problem for healthy adult chickens. Candidiasis and unsanitary, overcrowded conditions go together. Because the signs of candidiasis aren't apparent on the outside of the bird, a diagnostic laboratory usually diagnoses the disease during postmortem examination.

Dirty feeders or waterers are excellent places for the yeast to grow. Long-term antibiotic use also encourages yeast infections. Candidiasis isn't contagious between birds, but several birds living in the same filthy environment or exposed to antibiotics in feed or water can be affected at one time.

You can prevent candidiasis by having clean feeders, waterers, and coops, and by using antibiotics only when absolutely necessary. Candidiasis is treatable. If it's diagnosed in your flock, we suggest these treatment steps:

- Separate affected chickens from the rest of the flock so that they can't be picked on by flock mates.
- If you've been treating the chickens with antibiotics, stop it.
- Use a copper sulfate/vinegar solution in the drinking water (see the appendix for the recipe). You can find copper sulfate crystals at farm stores.
- Offer a probiotic (available at feed stores) or yogurt.
- Clean feeders and waterers daily.

Ringworm (Favus)

You've probably heard of (or had) ringworm, a fungal infection of the skin that people and pets can catch from each other. Chickens can also get ringworm and share the fungus with their flock keepers. (Here's a tip for word game players: *Favus* is the name for ringworm when it affects poultry.)

Ringworm usually appears as white scaly or crusty patches on the comb and the skin of the head and neck. The chicken may lose its feathers, typically starting at the base of the comb and progressing down the back of the neck. Other than the skin problem, affected chickens are usually healthy. The infection is contagious and spreads from bird to bird, and rarely, bird to human.

Any practicing veterinarian can do a skin scraping and fungal culture on a chicken to diagnose ringworm, the same way the fungal infection is diagnosed in other animals. If you have a chicken with favus, isolate it from the rest of the flock to prevent spreading the infection. People should wear gloves and wash their hands after handling the affected birds.

Rubbing the affected areas daily with athlete's foot ointment, or swabbing the spots with 2 percent iodine solution every other day should do the trick after about two weeks of treatment. Both medicines are available at any pharmacy. Ringworm fungus hates sunshine, so getting birds out of a dark shed and into the sunlight often cures favus without medicine.

Eyeing Diseases with Multiple or Mysterious Causes

For some chicken diseases, several events need to line up for the problem to occur. A combination of genetics, environment, and flock-management issues are common ingredients in a recipe for flock trouble. Sometimes the recipe is a secret, and we don't understand all the factors that add up to cause disease in chicken flocks. In this section, we describe a few multifactorial problems that you may face.

Broiler breakdowns

Some problems are unique to *broilers,* the strains of chickens that have been specifically designed by people for meat production. Backyard flock keepers can purchase day-old broiler chicks and raise them, usually up to 6 to 12 weeks of age, to supply home-grown meat for a family or small farm business.

Using intense selective breeding, poultry companies have created modern meat-type chicken strains that are vastly different from heritage breeds of poultry, such as their Plymouth Rock and Cornish breed ancestors. Modern broilers grow three times faster than old-fashioned breeds of chickens, and they need to eat only half of the feed to reach the same weight.

Explosive growth and super feed efficiency comes at price, however. Broilers grow too fast for their own good. Bones, joints, and internal organs barely (or can't) keep up with the rapid growth, and the result is a variety of these broiler breakdowns.

- **Ascites:** A broiler's heart may fail trying to pump blood to a rapidly growing body. The failing heart enlarges, and straw-colored fluid fills up the abdomen and lungs; this fluid build-up is called *ascites*. Birds with ascites may pant, even in cool weather, and their combs may have a bluish tinge.

   To lower the incidence of ascites, make sure your housing for broilers is well-ventilated. Dust and high ammonia levels increase cases of ascites in broiler flocks.

- **Leg problems:** Broilers can grow at a faster rate than their immature skeletal systems can support, leading to painful twisting or bowing of the legs or spine. Birds that are unwilling to get around because of leg pain or are unable to move well due to leg and back deformities may die of starvation, thirst, or trampling by flock mates.

- **Sudden death syndrome:** Healthy-looking broilers can flip over and die suddenly, expiring on their backs with a brief flurry of wing-flapping. You may think you've witnessed a fatal chicken heart attack. This event, known as *sudden death syndrome,* or *flip over disease,* is most commonly seen in broiler chickens between 2 and 4 weeks of age. Scientists don't understand the exact cause.

With a functional backyard lifespan of just a few months, broilers make terrible pet chickens. Broiler growers should be prepared to perform humane euthanasia for broken-down broilers.

Slowing that breakneck pace of growth, just a little, especially during the first three weeks of the growing period, can reduce the chances of ascites, leg problems, or sudden death syndrome in a batch of broilers. Feed restriction is the main method that you can use to slow growth. Here are two simple options for a broiler feed-restriction program:

- **Option 1:** Feed meals twice a day, rather than offering feed free-choice. Give the birds enough food so that they consume it all within three hours. No snacking between meals.

- **Option 2:** When the broilers are a week old, remove all feed from the pen every evening and put it back in the morning, 12 hours later. Do this every day until the birds are ready to be processed.

Other feed restriction methods, such as reduced-lighting programs and skip-a-day feeding, are more complicated and less practical in backyard settings. Whatever feed restriction program you use, make sure fresh water is always available. One last suggestion: Finely ground mash feed slows the greedy birds down a little, so it's a better choice than pelleted feed for broilers.

Bumblefoot (Pododermatitis)

Bumblefoot is the term used for any swelling of a toe or *foot pad* (the spongy bottom of the foot). The condition is an extremely common problem for older backyard hens. Chickens with bumblefoot usually limp, or in severe cases, don't use the leg at all due to pain. Bumblefoot starts as a minor injury, such as a bruise, puncture wound, scrape, or puncture wound, that you may not have noticed at first. Left untreated, the little wound can develop into a string of full-blown, deep-seated abscesses up and down the foot. Over time, the bacterial infection can destroy skin, tendon, or bone.

For every case of bumblefoot, there was not one, but a series of unfortunate events that led up to the problem. Here are some of the factors that set a bird up for a case of bumblefoot:

- Rough walking surfaces, such as concrete or gravel
- Bruised foot pads after jumping down from high perches
- Round or plastic perches
- Obesity
- Poor nutrition, especially high-carbohydrate diets (for example, too much scratch grain) or vitamin A deficiency
- Puncture wounds from splinters, protruding nails, or other sharp objects in the coop
- Wet bedding and cold weather

Compared to other parts of the body, a chicken's foot pads and toes don't get a lot of blood flow, especially in cold weather. Because of the lack of good blood flow to the area, healing an injured, inflamed, or infected foot is a slow, frustrating process.

Preventing bumblefoot is much more successful than treating bumblefoot. Optimum nutrition, good footing, and clean, dry bedding in the coop reduce the chances of foot sores leading to bumblefoot.

Good perch design for layer hens has been shown to reduce the number of sore feet in a flock. Use rectangular wooden perches, and 2-x-2-inch untreated hardwood lumber is ideal. To help hens land softly, space perches no more than 18 inches apart or above the floor.

Avian veterinarians have a lot of experience treating bumblefoot, because the condition occurs in all sorts of birds from pet parakeets to hunting falcons. Surgery to remove diseased tissue is the mainstay of bumblefoot treatment, along with bandaging and cleaning the wound. Antibiotic treatment is tricky; common bumblefoot-causing bacteria are resistant to many types of antibiotics. Even if the vet finds an antibiotic that the organism is sensitive to, a drug, the medication doesn't penetrate the low-blood flow foot tissue very well.

If consultation with a veterinarian isn't an option, you can try to treat some cases of bumblefoot at home, using these steps and being patient:

1. **Soak the affected foot daily for 15 minutes in a warm Epsom salt solution.**

   Softening a scabby wound is the goal so that you can peel away any scab and open the wound to clean it out.

   Wrap the chicken in a towel to calm and restrain it for daily bumblefoot wound cleaning.

2. **Flush the wound with a disinfectant solution and tweeze and trim away pus and any black, dead tissue.**

   A 20 mL syringe, a pair of forceps, and a sharp pair of toenail scissors are helpful tools. The appendix contains recipes for wound cleansing solutions. You can apply an antiseptic ointment, such as povidone-iodine or silver cream, after cleaning.

3. **Bandage the foot after cleaning the wound.**

   Figure 14-1 shows a bandaging method using swim noodle foam and self-cling bandaging tape. You can trim the section of swim noodle to fit the foot to take the pressure off the sore and allow easy access to the wound for daily cleaning.

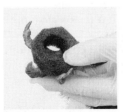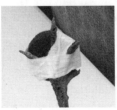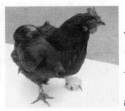

Photograph courtesy of Dave Gauthier, PhD

Figure 14-1: A bumblefoot dressing.

Crop problems: Sour crop and impactions

The bulge on the front of your chicken's neck is most likely normal. Chickens have a built-in doggie bag — the *crop,* which is a bulge in the esophagus where food treasures from foraging are saved for leisurely digestion another time. Sometimes, though, your chicken can develop problems where the crop won't empty properly, leading either to *sour crop* or *crop impaction:*

- ✔ **Sour crop:** It feels big and squishy, and a foul smell may come from the chicken's mouth.

- ✔ **Crop impaction:** It feels full and hard.

Either way, the chicken looks miserable and loses weight. An impaction may also extend downstream, to the gizzard, where you can't see the blockage. Possible causes of sour crop and crop impaction include:

- ✔ Gorging on long grass, hay, straw, wood chips, or sand, or eating strange things like string, baler twine, or plastic

- ✔ Diseases that slow down the movement of the gut, especially Marek's disease (see Chapter 12), egg peritonitis, or lead poisoning

- ✔ Damage to the gut from swallowed metal objects (hardware disease — see Chapter 11), or intestinal worms

You can be sure the bulge isn't a problem by checking the chicken in the morning, before she has eaten — the bulge should be gone then.

Some of the reasons for crop problems are grim: Marek's disease is fatal, and the prognosis for hardware disease, egg peritonitis, or severe gizzard impaction is awful. An experienced avian veterinarian can help determine the cause and offer surgical options, if it comes to that. The sooner you seek help, the better for the bird's chances of recovery. If consultation with an avian veterinarian isn't an option, you can focus on the potentially treatable causes with the following advice:

- ✔ Isolate the affected bird in a hospital pen and provide good nursing care, as we describe in Chapter 17. A cage with a wire floor and no bedding is preferable.

- ✔ Feed a commercial mash or crumbled diet and offer poultry grit made of crushed granite. Add 2 tablespoons of vinegar to each gallon of drinking water, and make sure the solution is fresh and constantly available.

✔ If the bird doesn't seem to be improving after a week of your good nursing care, consider euthanizing it rather than allowing it to waste away.

You may be tempted to give mineral oil or other liquid lubricants by mouth to break up an impaction. However, force-fed mineral oil or other liquids may end up in the bird's lungs, with a fatal result. Mineral oil doesn't help much to break up an impaction anyway (granite grit is more helpful than anything else you can give), so we don't recommend this practice.

You can prevent crop impactions in the following ways:

✔ Keep grass mowed short where chickens forage.

✔ Provide plenty of feeder space and always keep clean water available.

✔ Sweep the pen occasionally with a magnetic pick-up tool, which you can purchase at a hardware store for $20 or less.

✔ Be on the lookout for and remove old peeling paint from the flocks' domain, because it can be a source of toxic lead.

Gout and kidney stones

Gout in chickens isn't a single disease but a sign of dysfunctional kidneys. A long list of causes can lead to kidney disease, and high on the list are infections, nutritional imbalances, toxins, or water deprivation. If many birds in a flock are exposed to the same kidney-trashing circumstances, gout can kill a large proportion of a flock, maybe half of the birds.

Hens can do well with weak kidneys. They may look healthy and lay plenty of eggs, up to the point when kidney function is destroyed at 75 percent or more, and they can suddenly die without having shown any warning signs on the outside.

Inside a chicken with gout, however, the disease is obvious without a microscope. Healthy kidneys remove the waste products of the body's chemical reactions from the bloodstream. Diseased kidneys can't remove the wastes, so the waste products aren't removed and instead build up inside the body, deposited on and in various internal organs. The waste buildup creates a white, chalky coating to the internal organs. Tiny stones of the waste material can plug the urinary tract or accumulate in the joints.

You can prevent kidney damage and death from gout in your back-yard flock by sticking to these tips:

✔ **Don't feed layer diets to growing chickens.** Layer diets contain far too much calcium for chickens that aren't laying eggs, and the excess calcium is tough on the kidneys. (Refer to Chapter 6 for more on layer diets.)

✔ **Don't let the flock run out of water, ever.** Dehydrated kidneys work poorly; they need plenty of water to filter out body waste products.

✔ **Don't use baking soda long term in the chickens' drinking water.** Some flock keepers use baking soda (sodium bicarbonate) in drinking water to combat heat stress. Long-term use of baking soda can lead to gout, so we don't recommend the practice.

✔ **Don't use antibiotics unless absolutely necessary.** Some antibiotics can damage chicken kidneys.

You can attempt to treat gout in a flock with feed or water supplements that are mild acids. You can use vinegar in backyard flocks for this purpose, but the most effective dose and frequency haven't been determined yet. We suggest adding 2 tablespoons of vinegar per gallon of water and offering the solution as the flock's drinking water for 1 day each week.

Misfires of the reproductive tract

Damage to a hen's reproductive tract for any number of reasons, most frequently infections and tumors, can result in the egg-laying machinery going haywire. There is no treatment for the following three conditions:

✔ **False layer:** If the oviduct is blocked by a tumor or scar tissue, for example, yolks released from the ovary get dumped into the abdomen, rather than traveling down the oviduct in the normal route, and are gradually reabsorbed. The hen looks okay, but she doesn't lay eggs.

✔ **Internal layer:** In this case, the egg production line of the oviduct runs backwards, pushing developing eggs back up the line and dropping them inside the abdomen, rather than out the vent, leaving eggs in various stages of development floating around among the internal organs.

✔ **Sex reversal:** Every once in a while, a hen will turn into a rooster. At least, she'll act and look like a rooster, although she's still genetically female. She'll develop a crow, big comb and wattles, and long tail and neck feathers. (As far as we know, a rooster turning into a hen hasn't happened.) The causes of sex reversal are damage to the hen's single ovary, or growth of an abdominal tumor that produces testosterone.

Part IV

Your Chicken Repair Manual (and Advice for When to Close the Book)

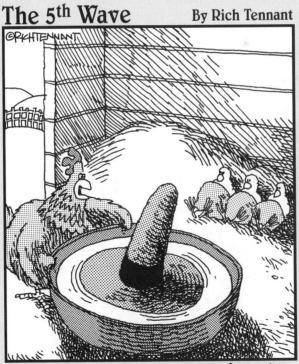

The 5th Wave   By Rich Tennant

@RICHTENNANT

"Alright, this should make everyone feel a little better. It's a bowl of my own, homemade chicken farmer soup. Sip it down carefully and watch for bones.

In this part...

We've met many flock keepers who are extremely self-reliant, or at least a little handy, either by character or out of necessity. This part will appeal to the do-it-yourselfers and come to the rescue of backyard flock keepers who suddenly find themselves in the role of first responder to chicken illnesses or injuries.

In this part, we show you how to vaccinate, medicate, collect samples, and repair injuries of chickens. When you need help or feel like you're getting in over your head, we have suggestions for experts to turn to. Finally, we deal with a subject that we believe all flock keepers should be prepared for — how to humanely euthanize a chicken when it's time to close the repair manual.

Chapter 15

Making a Diagnosis: Getting Advice or Going It Alone

....

....

*T*he first step in chicken repair is figuring out what's wrong — making a diagnosis. Without a diagnosis, treating a chicken or flock health problem is like playing darts blindfolded; you rarely hit a bull's-eye, and you may cause some damage if you miss by a wide margin. We hope that Chapters 7 through 10 troubleshoot and give you ideas of what's going on with a sick chicken. More than likely you're going to need some help to make an accurate diagnosis.

The good news: Several sources are available that you can turn to for help. We start this chapter by describing the professionals who are skilled at diagnosing health problems in chickens and how to find them. You can help your chicken-health advisor help you, by collecting useful samples for analysis. We provide tips on submitting good quality specimens to a diagnostic laboratory or a veterinarian.

But what if you can't find a veterinarian who sees chickens, and you're many miles from the closest laboratory? You can try to find the cause for a bird's demise by performing a postmortem at home. Doing so is easier (and less gruesome) than you may think. We take you through it step by step.

Finding Professionals Who Can Help You and Your Flock

What's your relationship with your chickens? Answering that question can give you a good idea which chicken-health advisor you need to find. Ask yourself the following questions to help you locate the right professional for your flock:

✔ Do you consider your chickens to be family members, with names and unique personalities? If so, you may want cutting-edge veterinary care for an individual pet chicken, provided by an avian specialist.

✔ Are your chickens a source of food or supplemental income for your family? In that case, spending a lot of money treating an individual sick chicken doesn't make sense. You may want to end a suffering bird's life humanely and to concentrate on overall flock health. Any veterinarian who is willing to treat poultry, veterinary diagnostic laboratories, and extension agents are valuable sources of advice for you.

If you're like most backyard flock keepers, your relationship is somewhere in the middle of the spectrum of pets to food, and you keep chickens as good companions who return your investment of care with fresh eggs. You have some difficult choices to make, balancing the welfare of your pets with the cost of treatment and food-safety concerns.

Hens are different from all other family pets, because they produce food for people on a daily basis. When you're discussing treatment plans with your chicken health advisor, always keep in mind that chickens are food-producing animals (even if a chicken lives in an apartment, wears a diaper, and sleeps in a bed!). Any medication given to a chicken ends up in the eggs or meat, so to protect human health, laws restrict which treatments can be given to chickens.

The following sections discuss the different types of veterinarians and other professionals who you may turn to for help.

Locating a chicken vet

You won't find a chicken vet on every corner. Most U.S. veterinary students get very little training in chicken medicine, and they don't feel confident treating chickens when they graduate. A few vets take extra courses in caring for pet birds and other exotic pets, and a few others focus especially on the health of commercial food-producing poultry. To help you find a veterinarian who has knowledge and interest in chicken health, we describe the roles of each type of professional.

Avian veterinarians

For state-of the-art care of an individual pet chicken, an avian veterinarian is the best choice. State-of-the-art care, of course, isn't inexpensive. Avian veterinarians have a special interest in the medical and surgical treatment of birds — all types of birds, from finches to ostriches. They may work in private practice, veterinary colleges, zoos, and wildlife rehabilitation facilities. Tools at the disposal of an avian veterinarian include blood work, X-rays, anesthesia, surgery, and intensive-care equipment.

Some avian veterinarians complete additional formal training after veterinary school to become board-certified specialists in avian practice. You can recognize a board-certified avian specialist by the *Diplomate ABVP — Avian Practice* printed after his or her name.

The Association of Avian Veterinarians maintains an online database of member veterinarians that you can search by location. Find an avian veterinarian near you at www.aav.org/search/index.php.

General practitioners

A few practicing veterinarians (especially those who keep chickens themselves) have an interest in treating chickens and helping backyard flock keepers. These general practitioners are a rare (some say endangered) breed of animal doctors. They may not have received much formal training in chicken health, but they generally have some in-the-trenches experience with chicken illnesses and, more importantly, enthusiasm for chicken keeping.

If you can find such a person, any licensed veterinarian with an interest in treating chickens is a great resource for practical advice, but not necessarily cutting-edge care. General practitioners who like to see chickens usually spend most of their time treating animals like dogs, cats, cattle, or horses, and are happy to see a poultry patient once in a while. Some research, trust, and trial and error from both you and your vet with a chicken interest can build a successful relationship.

We don't know of any professional organization or official list for veterinarians who are willing and able to see backyard chickens, so you need to talk to fellow flock keepers to find the right vet. Online chicken-keeping discussion forums are a good place to start.

Exploring other sources of help

We often hear the comment that flock keepers can't find a veterinarian who is willing to treat or knows anything about chickens. If you feel this way, you can refer to the following options for finding a chicken health advisor in your area.

Poultry vets: Not often accessible to backyard flock keepers

Poultry veterinarians know chickens; they're the experts when it comes to chicken disease and chicken flock health. Many poultry veterinarians spend several years in additional training after veterinary school to become specialists in the diagnosis and management of health problems of birds used for food.

Unfortunately, poultry vets aren't easily accessible by backyard flock keepers. Many poultry vets are independent consultants or employed as technical specialists for large companies associated with the poultry industry. These industry vets usually won't visit backyard chicken flocks out of concern that they could carry a disease back to a large commercial poultry flock. On the other hand, poultry vets who work for universities can visit and often do help backyard flock keepers.

The primary goal of poultry vets is to prevent disease in a flock. If a health problem does sneak into a flock, poultry vets make recommendations for managing or treating the entire flock to minimize the effects of the illness and the economic loss for the producer. Generally, they don't treat individual birds.

If you have a dream of selling eggs or meat from your small farm operation, a poultry vet is an invaluable adviser to help you keep your flock healthy, productive, and on the right side of food safety laws. Get in touch with the extension office, veterinary school, or veterinary diagnostic laboratory closest to you, and ask for names of poultry vets working in your area.

Extension agents

The Cooperative Extension System is a nationwide educational network in the United States. Each state has one or more extension offices connected with a university, staffed by experts who provide practical, research-based information to farmers, small business owners, consumers, and young people through the 4-H youth development program.

In recent years, this system has shrunk; fewer offices and fewer extension agents, who must wear multiple hats, serve more and more people. At one time, many extension offices had an agent who specialized in livestock and poultry production. If you're lucky, you live in a state that still has a poultry specialist working in an extension office. If not, your local extension agents are helpful resources regardless of their areas of expertise, because they're well connected in their communities and can probably find an answer to your question or refer you to someone who can help, possibly a colleague in another state.

You can find an extension office near you, and find extension service publications about poultry health at www.extension.org.

National Poultry Improvement Plan

The National Poultry Improvement Plan (NPIP) is a cooperative industry, state, and federal program started in the 1930s to eliminate pullorum disease, which was rampant at the time and killed many chicks. Now, pullorum disease is nearly extinct in chicken flocks in the United States.

Backyard flock keepers can participate in the NPIP and have their flocks inspected, tested, and certified pullorum disease–free by NPIP representatives. In most states, joining the program and having the tests performed doesn't cost much. Depending on the state where you live, other flock certification tests, such as avian influenza or *Mycoplasma gallisepticum* (MG) testing, may also be available to you.

If you want to ship hatching eggs or chicks across state lines or take chickens to shows in other states, you'll want to be an NPIP participant to make it easier for you to meet state animal-import requirements. Find your state's NPIP representative and names of participating flock keepers at www.aphis.usda.gov/animal_health/animal_dis_spec/poultry/participants.shtml.

Poultry nutritionists

Feed mills work with poultry nutritionists to come up with the recipes for their chicken diets. If you have a question about chicken nutrition, your feed supplier can put you in touch with the feed mill or poultry nutritionist who prepared the feed that you use. You can also look up the contact information for the nutritionists on your brand's website.

Poultry science departments at universities

If you have questions about achieving optimum egg production or managing meat-type chickens for maximum growth and feed efficiency, a poultry scientist working in a university animal science department is definitely the go-to person. Poultry scientists are also excellent consultants for troubleshooting incubation and hatching problems and answering your questions about chicken genetics and diseases.

We list U.S. poultry science departments in Chapter 1.

State veterinarians

Each U.S. state has a state veterinarian who oversees animal disease control and animal welfare in that state. The state veterinarian's office regulates the movement of chickens across state lines, makes sure that poultry at shows and fairs are healthy, and investigates outbreaks of chicken disease.

You can find your state veterinarian at this website: `www.usaha.org/Portals/6/StateAnimalHealthOfficials.pdf`. Contact your state veterinarian if you have questions about moving chickens in and out of the state, or to report an outbreak of chicken disease.

Veterinary diagnostic laboratories

A network of veterinary diagnostic laboratories provides services to animal owners and their veterinarians throughout the United States. These laboratories are often connected with a state university and/or government agriculture department. Laboratory staff can run blood tests, examine tissue samples, and perform postmortems on animals as small as mice and as large as elephants.

Animal owners usually work with a diagnostic laboratory through their veterinarians, but most laboratories accept samples submitted directly by owners. In many states, the state department of agriculture subsidizes the costs of poultry tests and postmortem examinations as a service to the farming community. This deal is great for backyard flock keepers, and you may find the fees to be surprisingly low.

Although a laboratory's staff has amazing skills for making a diagnosis of animal disease, they can't give treatment advice or provide clinical care the way a licensed veterinarian can.

You can find lists of veterinary diagnostic laboratories by visiting the American Association of Veterinary Laboratory Diagnosticians site at `www.aavld.org/accreditation1` or the National Animal Health Laboratory Network site at `www.aphis.usda.gov/animal_health/nahln/labs.shtml`.

Collecting Samples for Your Chicken-Health Advisor

If you're a do-it-yourself type, you can easily collect and submit some types of samples to your veterinarian or diagnostic laboratory. Dead birds and samples of droppings or external parasites are specimens commonly submitted by flock keepers. The following sections discuss some different instances where you may need to submit samples for testing.

Submitting a chicken for postmortem examination

When you have a chicken die mysteriously, you're probably curious and want some closure to determine the chicken's cause of death. As a result, you can submit the chicken's body for a postmortem. A chicken *postmortem* is an excellent tool to monitor the whole flock's health. For example, a postmortem is the only way you'll find out for certain that Marek's disease is in your flock.

 Submitting a dead chicken to a veterinary diagnostic laboratory can provide you with a tremendous amount of information about your flock. However it can also be a tremendous waste of time, if a carcass isn't in good condition when it arrives at the laboratory. When you submit a (useful) dead chicken, stick to these steps:

1. **Immediately cool the bird's body after death and keep it cool during transport to the lab.**

   Double-bag the carcass (kitchen-size trash bags work well) and place it in a refrigerator or in a cooler with ice. Don't freeze the carcass. Dead birds that have been lying around for just a couple of hours in hot weather are probably already too badly decomposed to be useful. Don't waste your time (or the lab's time) with old carcasses.

2. **Call the laboratory.**

   Get instructions for dropping off or shipping the carcass. A lab usually has a designated reception area for dead animals. You may be able to ship a carcass in a cooler with ice packs; ask the lab staff for packaging and shipping instructions.

3. **Be prepared to discuss details about your flock and about the bird's behavior before death.**

   You'll be asked about the size of your flock, the age of the chicken, any signs of illness prior to death, where the bird came from, and whether it was vaccinated against any disease. The veterinary pathologist will find these and other details helpful for solving the case. The flock notebook we mention in Chapter 7 comes in handy here.

4. **Discuss with laboratory staff how far you're willing to go to get a precise diagnosis.**

   The veterinary pathologist doing the postmortem evaluation may be able to get a good idea of the cause of death just from a visual inspection of the carcass. Often additional tests (with additional expense) are necessary, such as looking at tissue samples under a microscope or conducting tests to identify bacteria or viruses.

Many diagnostic laboratories accept live, sick chickens and euthanize them for you, providing the freshest, most useful specimens
for postmortem examination. Ask the lab if this option is available.

Collecting specimens for parasite identification

If you suspect a parasite is bugging your chickens on the outside
or inside, you can collect and submit samples for external and
internal parasite identification and submit them for testing. These
sections explain what to collect and how to do so.

Trapping external parasite specimens

To identify parasites that you find crawling on your chickens, tape
preps and digital photography are two methods you can use to
submit the bugs for identification. We explain the two methods here:

- ✔ **Tape prep:** You can do a *tape prep* to catch lice and mites for
  identification. Press short pieces of cellophane tape onto the
  chicken's skin where you see the unidentified crawling objects
  and their debris. The tape will trap and hold the parasites
  during transport to your veterinarian or diagnostic laboratory. An empty pill vial is an ideal container for shipping the
  tape pieces.

- ✔ **Digital photography:** Lights, camera, action. Groom an infested
  chicken with a comb while the bird is standing on a piece of
  white paper. Dump any parasites that fall onto the paper into a
  sealable plastic bag and place the bag in a freezer for 15 minutes
  to slow down the bugs. Take a close-up photograph of the chilled
  parasites on the white paper background with the macro mode
  of a digital camera. Take several images, and e-mail the best
  images to a laboratory for identification. Contact a veterinary
  diagnostic laboratory or your local extension agent who can
  guide you to a pest identification laboratory.

Scooping poop for internal parasite ID

If you're concerned that internal parasites are causing problems
for your flock, a veterinarian's office or diagnostic laboratory can
examine droppings under a microscope and look for the parasites
or their eggs. You can collect poop samples from individual birds
kept in separate cages for a few hours, or you can collect a composite sample from the flock overnight.

To collect a composite sample of droppings from a flock, follow
these steps:

1. **Place newspaper or brown kraft paper under coop perches in the evening, after the chickens have gone to roost.**

2. **In the morning, scrape several poops off different areas on the paper into a container with a tight-fitting lid, and stir the sample before sealing the container.**

   Each container should represent about five to ten birds; larger flocks require several containers. Plastic yogurt containers, with the lid taped closed, or large pill vials are perfect containers for this purpose.

3. **Bag the containers in large plastic zipper lock bags and keep the samples in the refrigerator until it's time to deliver them.**

   Make sure you label the container and warn the household what's in it.

Performing a DIY Postmortem

Imagine yourself in this scenario: One of your chickens has died, and you don't know why — nothing is obvious on the outside of the bird. You haven't found a local veterinarian to help you with your chickens, and the nearest veterinary diagnostic laboratory is several hours away by car. Driving there with one dead chicken isn't practical.

You call fellow flock keepers, post a note on an online backyard chicken discussion group, or call your extension agent. "My chicken has died. What could be the cause? Is the rest of my flock at risk?" If blank looks could be transmitted virtually, or over the phone, blank looks are what you get.

Without more clues, your advisors can only speculate about the cause of death. You need to look inside the bird to get those clues. In this section, we guide you through a postmortem examination, more formally called a *necropsy* when it's performed on an animal.

A necropsy, even a very thorough one performed by an expert, won't always reveal the cause of death, but you never know if you don't look.

Performing a necropsy on a single dead chicken is a do-it-yourself job. Diagnosing a flock die-off isn't. If you're losing many birds to illness, don't perform a postmortem yourself. Double-bag the dead birds, store them in a refrigerator or in a cooler with ice, and call your state veterinarian for help right away.

If you're going to perform a postmortem, these sections can help make the process easier.

Gathering equipment and getting started

In order to perform a postmortem, you need the following equipment:

- ✔ A washable table in a well-lit place
- ✔ Water, soap, and towels
- ✔ A pair of heavy-duty scissors such as kitchen shears
- ✔ Disposable exam gloves
- ✔ Something to take notes on

Before diving in, examine the bird's outside. Look at the head for signs of discharge from the eyes, nostrils, or mouth. Judge the bird's body condition, using the scoring system in Chapter 7. Check for scabs on the combs, face, and wattles. Inspect the feathers and peek at the vent area for signs of lice or mite infestations.

Dunk the carcass in a bucket of soapy water before you start the internal examination. Doing so can keep feathers from flying everywhere and getting in your way.

Necropsying a chicken, step by step

You may want to review chicken anatomy (which we present in Chapter 2) before you make your first cut. As you perform the steps, jot down notes about anything that puzzles you during the necropsy. Describe the color, size, texture, and location of the things you saw in simple terms (for example, "many small white spots on the liver") so that you can look up your findings later or describe them to your chicken health advisor. The following steps help you with the internal examination.

Starting the postmortem

When you're ready to begin the postmortem, stick to these steps:

1. **To position the bird, place the bird on its back with the legs toward you.**

2. **Grasp both legs and push them down toward the table to flatten the legs away from the body.**

   The hip joints will pop when you've done this correctly.

3. **To open the abdomen and chest cavity, pick up the skin over the abdomen with your fingers to make a tent and cut through the skin with your scissors, as shown in Figure 15-1.**

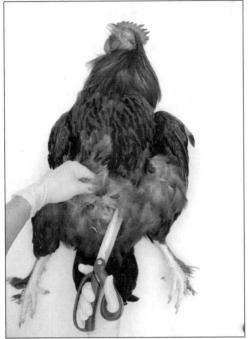

Photograph courtesy of Dave Gauthier, PhD

Figure 15-1: Making the first cut to open the abdomen.

4. **Using your hands, peel the skin up toward the head to expose the breast.**

   Look at the breast muscle. Is the keel bone prominent because the breast muscle is shrunken? Is the breast muscle pale or bruised?

5. **Cut through the ribs and muscle on the sides of the keel.**

   Grasp the lower point of the keel and pull upward to lift the breast and expose the internal organs in the chest and abdomen. See Figure 15-2.

Examining and removing the internal organs

When you're ready to inspect the internal organs, keep following these steps:

1. **Identify the liver, which is a large, dark red organ.**

   The normal-sized liver shouldn't extend past the tip of the breast. Check the liver for white or yellow spots and lumps that may indicate infection or tumors.

2. **Make sure the abdominal cavity is free of fluid and looks clean.**

   Blood or blood clots in the abdomen can signal *fatty liver hemorrhagic syndrome* (see Chapter 11). Gunk that looks like scrambled egg floating in the abdomen is a sign of *egg peritonitis* (see Chapter 12). Lots of clear, yellowish-tinged fluid indicates a condition called *ascites* (see Chapter 14).

3. **Try to find the air sacs.**

   Normal air sacs look like soap bubbles or clear cellophane wrap. Cloudy or gunky air sacs are a sign of a lower respiratory tract infection.

4. **Remove the liver, gall bladder, and spleen.**

   The spleen is a round, reddish organ located near the stomachs, and the gall bladder is nestled in the center of the liver — a little green discoloration in that area is normal.

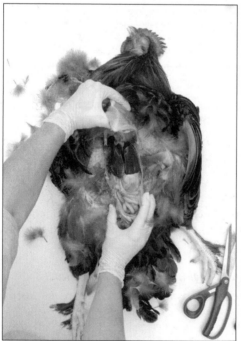

Photograph courtesy of Dave Gauthier, PhD

Figure 15-2: Lift the breast to reveal the chest and abdominal cavities.

5. **Remove the heart, which is encased in a thin, almost see-through membrane.**

   Cut through this membrane to view the heart's outside surface. A little clear fluid between the membranous heart sac and the heart is normal. A lot of fluid in the sac or a cloudy, rough surface on the outside of the heart indicates an infection.

6. **Find the place where the esophagus enters the stomachs (the *proventriculus* and gizzard).**

   Cut through the esophagus. Lift the guts — the stomachs, intestines, and ceca — out of the abdomen as you trim the thin membrane that holds them inside the abdomen. Cut through the large intestine where it exits the body at the vent, in order to free the whole package of guts from the abdomen. Set the digestive tract (see Figure 15-3) aside for a closer look later (see Step 10).

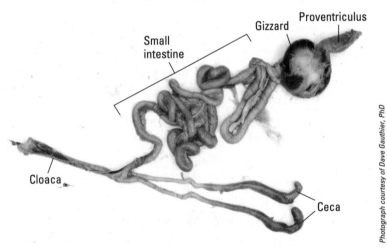

Figure 15-3: Lay out the digestive tract to identify the parts.

7. **Inspect the organs close to the backbone.**

   The kidneys are embedded along each side of the backbone. A normal pair of kidneys is elongated, dark reddish-brown, and symmetrical. Feel the kidneys, and cut into them to look for crunchy, whitish kidney stones.

8. **Find the reproductive organs.**

   In roosters, a pair of whitish bean-shaped testicles is located above the kidneys. In hens, the left ovary, which looks like a bunch of orangey-yellow grapes, is positioned on top of the left kidney. (The right ovary doesn't develop in female chickens.) You may find an egg under construction within the oviduct.

9. **Using your fingers, tease the lungs away from the ribcage.**

   They should be light pink and spongy.

10. **Go back to the digestive tract that you removed earlier (see Step 6) and, starting at the stomach end, cut along the entire length of the digestive tract toward the cloaca at the vent end.**

    You'll be cutting through the proventriculus, gizzard, and small intestine. Also cut open each of the two ceca and lay them open. The gizzard is muscular and tough to cut, and it's normal to find grit (small stones) inside.

11. **Rinse the lining of the stomachs, intestines, and ceca with water to flush away the contents for a better view.**

    Look for bleeding and thickened red patches in the lining of the gut that are tip-offs for coccidiosis (see Chapter 13). You may also see intestinal worms waving at you.

12. **Search for the *bursa of Fabricius*.**

    In a chicken less than 4 months old, you may be able to find this important organ of the growing bird's immune system when you cut through the cloaca at the end of the digestive tract.

    A normal bursa is a small, grape-like pouch with a wrinkled, cream-colored interior. *Infectious bursal disease* causes redness and jelly-like swelling of the bursa.

Looking inside the head and neck

To inspect the head and neck in your postmortem exam, keep following these steps:

1. **Turn the bird around to face you.**

   Use your scissors and cut through the corner of the mouth. Keep cutting through the skin down the neck toward the chest, to expose the trachea, esophagus, and the crop, as shown in Figure 15-4. The *trachea* (windpipe) is the stiff tube that looks a little like a drinking straw. The flat, pink tube running alongside the trachea is the esophagus, which carries swallowed food to the stomachs. If you follow along the esophagus to where it enters the chest cavity, you find an enlargement, or pouch, in the esophagus, which is the chicken's crop.

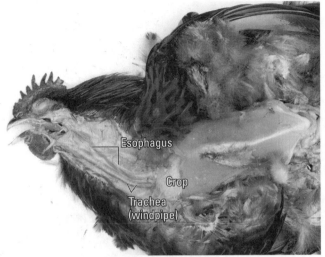

Figure 15-4: Cut along the neck to show the trachea, esophagus, and crop.

2. **Cut open the esophagus along its length, all the way down to the crop.**

   Look for food or indigestible stuff that the chicken shouldn't have eaten. You can rinse the crop with water to get a clearer view of the lining. A roughened, towel-like appearance of the inside of the crop is a sign of a yeast infection called candidiasis (see Chapter 14).

3. **View the lining inside the trachea by cutting it lengthwise.**

   Blood, cheesy material, or lots of mucous are evidence of a respiratory infection. If a chicken has a gapeworm infection, you find the reddish worms here, attached to the lining of the trachea.

Inspecting joints and nerves and finishing

To take the finishing steps of your postmortem, you want to inspect the joints and nerves:

1. **Turn the bird around to its original position with its feet toward you.**

2. **Find the large *sciatic nerve* that runs along the inside of each upper thigh, under the thigh muscle.**

   See Figure 15-5 for normal chicken sciatic nerves. The nerves should be smooth and symmetrical. An enlargement of a sciatic nerve is one indication of Marek's disease (see Chapter 12).

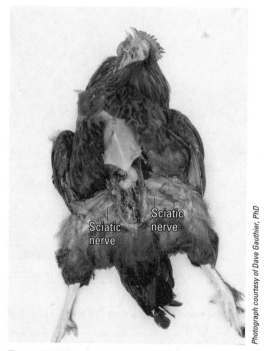

Photograph courtesy of Dave Gauthier, PhD

Figure 15-5: Normal sciatic nerves in a chicken.

3. **Inspect the leg joints for swellings.**

   Cut the leg joints open with your scissors. The joints' surface should be smooth with some clear, sticky joint fluid. Blood, pus, or cloudy fluid in the joint is a sign of infection.

4. **Properly dispose of the carcass and tissues.**

   We provide carcass disposal suggestions in Chapter 18. Used paper towels and gloves can go in the trash, but make sure animal scavengers (including your live chickens) can't get into the trash receptacle.

5. **Clean and disinfect the table, your scissors, and your hands.**

Chapter 16

Medicating and Vaccinating Chickens

In This Chapter

▶ Recognizing that any chicken is a potential food-producing animal

▶ Deciding whether you really need to use an antibiotic or vaccine

▶ Getting the stuff into the chicken and not all over you

*D*eciding whether to use medications or vaccinations for chickens is often more difficult than the nuts and bolts of actually administering them. Medications and vaccinations can help chickens survive illness and feel better faster, but they also have the potential to cause harm to the patient or to people who eat eggs or meat from treated chickens.

Germs and parasites can develop resistance to antibiotic or deworming treatments, so flock keepers should use those important medications only when necessary to help preserve their effectiveness. You have several options for administering medications or vaccinations you decide to use, and we take you through those techniques step by step in this chapter.

Grasping the Link between Drugs and Food-Producing Animals

In the eyes of many people, and in the eyes of U.S. food safety officials, chickens are food-producing animals, and strict rules limit how flock keepers and veterinarians can medicate them. It doesn't matter if a hen's day job is pampered pet, movie star, or full-time professional egg-layer; if she is a member of the species *Gallus gallus domesticus* (the domesticated fowl), she's a food-producing animal and the food animal drug laws apply to her.

Banned from use in food animals

If you're curious about the drugs prohibited from use for food animals, visit www.farad.org/eldu/prohibit.asp to see the list.

What's so terrible about these drugs that they're banned from use in food-producing animals? Are they super-toxic for animals, or deadly for people who eat meat, milk, or eggs from animals treated with the drugs? No, except in very rare instances or freak events, serious immediate harm isn't the issue. Here are the reasons that some drugs are banned from use in food animals:

✔ The drug is suspected or known to cause cancer in people or animals.

✔ The drug causes adverse reactions in a few people who are particularly sensitive to it.

✔ The antibiotic is very important for treating serious infections in people, and public health officials want to reserve the antibiotic for life-saving treatment. Any use of antibiotics, anywhere, anytime, for people or animals, has the potential to create drug-resistant superbugs. Reducing the use of important antibiotics may put off the inevitable — development of antibiotic resistant germs — a little bit longer.

We don't cover this topic because we think the chicken-drug police are peering over every backyard fence (you can safely say food-safety officials have other priorities). We discuss it because there are good reasons for the rules that limit drug use for food-producing animals. After all, who wants their order of two eggs over-easy to come with a side of antibiotics? Any medication given to chickens has the potential to wind up in eggs or meat. We lay out the facts so you can make an informed decision about medicating your chickens.

Flock keepers can use medications they purchase over the counter to treat their chickens as long as they follow the directions on the label. Any use of a medication in a way that isn't listed on the label is called *extra-label use*. Here are a few examples of extra-label drug use:

✔ Giving a cattle dewormer to a chicken for treatment of intestinal parasites.

✔ Giving an antibiotic for seven days when the label reads, "Treat for five days."

✔ Giving a medication by mouth, when the label indicates the drug should be given by injection under the skin.

According to U.S. Food and Drug Administration (FDA) regulations, extra-label drug use in food-producing animals by anyone other than a licensed veterinarian is illegal. Some drugs are completely prohibited for food-producing animals — even veterinarians can't prescribe them for chickens. Examples of drugs on the no-no list are popular dog and cat antibiotics enrofloxacin (Baytril) and cephalexin (Keflex). Also, no one (including veterinarians) is allowed to use medicated feed in a way that isn't spelled out on the feed label.

Following the extra-label drug rules set by the FDA, your veterinarian can prescribe medications for your chickens. Here is a summary of those rules:

- ✔ You and your vet must have a *valid veterinarian-client-patient relationship.* This relationship means that your veterinarian is personally acquainted with you and your chickens. Long-distance relationships (telephone or Internet consultations) don't count; they aren't considered valid.

- ✔ Your veterinarian must provide you with directions for using the drug and keep records about the prescription for two years.

- ✔ If the drug will be used for meat or egg-producing chickens, the veterinarian must advise you about a *withdrawal time,* which is the number of days that people must avoid eating eggs or meat from chickens after you stop the treatment. See the nearby sidebar for more information on withdrawal time.

Calculating a withdrawal time

Your veterinarian must provide you with a withdrawal time when prescribing a drug for chickens, in order to protect people from eating eggs or meat with drug residues. For many medications, though, information about how long a medication may remain in a treated chicken's eggs doesn't exist, so a veterinarian must make a best guess and add some time as a safety factor.

Considering the time it takes for a hen's body to make an egg (several weeks from start to finish), any egg laid eight weeks or longer after a hen stopped receiving a drug is highly unlikely to contain traces of it. A two-month egg discard time is wise if the actual withdrawal time isn't known. For some drugs, research has shown that they don't hang around that long, and a shorter withdrawal period is okay for those medications.

The Food Animal Residue Avoidance Databank (FARAD) is an excellent resource to help your veterinarian figure out a withdrawal time. If your veterinarian hasn't heard of FARAD, ask him or her to go to https://cafarad.ucdavis.edu/ FARMWeb/. Your vet can submit a question about withdrawal information for drugs or chemicals used for chickens and receive an answer from FARAD staff, usually within 72 hours.

Deciding to Use Antibiotics

An antibiotic can be a magic wand for a sick chicken, but wave that wand too often, and the magic can wear out. A consequence of using an antibiotic is the possibility of creating antibiotic resistant germs. You can use the following tips to help you decide when and how to use an antibiotic.

- ✔ **Focus on prevention.** Preventing disease through good biosecurity and keeping the flock clean, comfortable, and well fed is cheaper, safer, and more effective than treating disease. *Biosecurity* practices are things you do routinely to prevent harmful organisms from invading your flock. We give practical tips for backyard biosecurity in Chapter 4.

- ✔ **Before you reach for an antibiotic, try TLC.** Chickens are amazingly resilient creatures. Sometimes a chicken just needs a little help from her friends in order to heal herself. A warm, dry place away from the harassment of flock mates, good food, and a vitamin and electrolyte supplement may be just what the doctor ordered, instead of an antibiotic. We give advice for sick chicken TLC in Chapter 17.

- ✔ **Read the label and call your vet.** Following the label directions ensures that people won't be exposed to drug residues in eggs or meat. If you have questions about an over-the-counter or prescription medication, your veterinarian can advise you on whether to use the medication and how to do it safely.

- ✔ **Treat the smallest number of animals and treat only as long as needed.** Don't medicate the whole flock for one sick chicken. Unnecessary mass-medication and long, drawn-out treatments give germs plenty of time and opportunity to develop resistance.

- ✔ **Keep records.** If you don't jot down what, when, and who you medicated, you'll be asking yourself later, "Now when did I start that medicine? Did I give it to this brown hen, or that one?" Treated chickens should carry ID. You can purchase numbered or colored leg bands from poultry supply companies. In a pinch, you can use plastic zip ties, which are available at any hardware store, as leg bands.

Answering the Big Question: To Vaccinate or Not to Vaccinate?

When you have a small backyard flock, you probably wonder whether you should vaccinate. The bottom line is that vaccination probably isn't necessary for most backyard flocks. If your flock is a *closed* flock — if chickens don't come and go from your place — the risk that a vaccine-preventable disease will invade your flock is small.

However, in some situations, you can save a flock and prevent chicken suffering and death if you vaccinate your chickens. You should consider vaccination if any of these conditions is true for your flock:

✔ You take chickens to poultry shows and bring them back home.

✔ You buy chickens from auctions, poultry shows, or other places where birds gather, and add them to your existing flock.

✔ Your flock has had a vaccine-preventable disease problem in the past.

✔ Outbreaks of a vaccine-preventable chicken disease occur in the area where you live.

Reviewing vaccines for backyard chickens

Three vaccines are commonly used by backyard flock keepers to protect their chickens from disease: fowl pox, Marek's disease, and infectious laryngotracheitis (ILT) vaccines. Table 16-1 shows the method used to give each of the three vaccines and the recommended vaccination schedule.

Table 16-1 Vaccines to Consider for Small Chicken Flocks

Disease	Method	Age at First Vaccination	Booster Age
Fowl pox	Injected in the skin of the wing web	1–4 weeks	8–12 weeks
Infectious laryngo-tracheitis (ILT)	Eyedrop	4 weeks and older	yearly
Marek's disease	Injected under the skin	1 day	none

Fowl pox vaccine

Mosquitoes and fowl pox go together (refer to Chapter 12), and they're both regular, unwelcome summertime visitors for some flocks. Vaccination before mosquito season kicks off each year can protect your young birds from the misery of fowl pox. You can purchase fowl pox vaccine from veterinary supply companies. Read on for a description of the wing web vaccination technique used to give fowl pox vaccine; it's a fairly simple job. (Read the "Wing web stab" section later in this chapter for more information.)

Marek's disease vaccine

Marek's disease is a sad, common, and deadly chicken disease that causes tumors and paralysis; we discuss it in more detail in Chapter 12. After a flock has a case of Marek's disease, the disease sticks around for good, because the virus that causes it can linger for many months in dust and feather dander. Vaccination against Marek's disease is a valuable tool to protect each new generation or addition to that infected flock. Marek's disease vaccination doesn't prevent chicks from becoming infected with the virus, but it does a good job (not a perfect job) of preventing the virus from causing disease.

For a small fee, many hatcheries will vaccinate your mail-order, day-old chicks against Marek's disease. We can't think of a serious drawback to having a hatchery vaccinate chicks, so take the hatchery up on this offer. If you hatch your own chicks, you can purchase Marek's disease vaccine from veterinary supply companies and give it yourself to newly hatched chicks. Read the later section "Under the skin" for a description of how the vaccine is given under the skin.

Infectious laryngotracheitis (ILT) vaccine

As we discuss in Chapter 12, ILT is a nasty respiratory virus that affects adult chickens. Show birds are particularly at risk for picking up the virus from poultry shows and bringing it home to share with the rest of the flock. Annual vaccination against ILT, at least 30 days before show season starts, is something that people who keep exhibition flocks should consider for their valuable birds.

Use only *tissue culture origin* (TCO) ILT vaccine for your flock. Two types of ILT vaccine are available for backyard flock keepers to purchase: TCO and *chicken embryo origin* (CEO) vaccine. The TCO ILT vaccine has been proven to be very safe, but the CEO ILT vaccine has been known to create the disease it was intended to prevent.

Other vaccines

Other poultry vaccines, such as shots against infectious bronchitis, infectious coryza, Newcastle disease, or fowl cholera are available, but we don't recommend them unless the disease has been diagnosed in your flock or in your neighborhood. Your veterinarian or veterinary diagnostic laboratory can help you decide if vaccination is a good idea for your flock.

Poultry vaccines: Not small flock-friendly

One big barrier to the use of vaccines in small flocks is the way that they're packaged and sold. Because large commercial chicken farmers use most of the poultry vaccine produced, the vaccinations are packaged in hundreds or thousands of doses, which isn't cost-effective or convenient for vaccinating small numbers of birds. Vaccines don't keep, so small flock owners have to resign themselves to paying for and throwing out hundreds of doses.

Also, cutting-edge poultry vaccines are stored and administered with specialized equipment, so unless you have a tank of liquid nitrogen or an egg-injection machine, you probably won't be using the most up-to-date poultry vaccine technology.

Backyard flock ownership is booming, and small flock owners are savvy consumers who want the best for their chickens. Maybe it's time for small flock owners to unite and encourage vaccine companies to make and package vaccines that are practical for small flocks.

Vaccinating successfully

Deciding whether to give shots is just the first dilemma for backyard flock keepers to solve in the vaccination conundrum. After you opt to give shots to your chickens, you need to give the right stuff, at the right time, and in the right place, in order for your efforts to be effective at preventing disease in the flock. Here are some pointers for vaccinating chickens successfully:

- ✔ **Vaccination is no substitute for good biosecurity and keeping the flock clean, comfortable, and well-fed.** Vaccines can't protect birds when they're overwhelmed by life in a filthy environment teeming with viruses and bacteria. Refer to Chapter 5 for creating a clean and relaxing environment for your flock.

- ✔ **Vaccinate before the chicken is exposed to the disease.** A vaccine works by stimulating the chicken's own immune system to fight specific diseases, and the immune system needs time (usually at least two weeks) to make antibodies and build defenses. Vaccinating for a disease after the chicken is already sick isn't helpful.

- ✔ **Keep vaccines cool.** Vaccines sent by mail should arrive in an insulated container with ice packs that are still cool. If the vaccine is warm when it arrives, call the supplier. Put the vaccine in a refrigerator as soon as you receive it, and keep it there until you use it. After you mix the vaccine in preparation for using it, keep it on an ice pack.

Treating organic backyard chickens

In the United States, chicken meat or eggs can be labeled *organic* if the food was produced according to National Organic Program (NOP) standards, which you can read at www.ams.usda.gov/nop/. Other countries have similar organic programs with slightly different rules.

If you produce less than $5,000 worth of food per year from your small farm and you follow NOP standards, you don't have to be certified to label your products organic. If your farm produces more than $5,000 worth of food per year, an NOP agent must inspect and certify your operation in order for you to sell certified organic food.

In a nutshell, U.S. organic chicken meat and egg producers follow the animal health and welfare standards of the NOP. They feed 100 percent organic feed to their chickens and provide them access to the outdoors. To be labeled organic, chicken meat and eggs can come only from chickens that haven't received antibiotics or other medications listed as prohibited in the lengthy NOP National List of Allowed and Prohibited Substances. Here are some other rules that people who want to raise chickens organically should know about vaccinating and medicating them:

✔ Vaccination is allowed and encouraged to keep organic livestock healthy.

✔ Medication can't be withheld from organic livestock in order to preserve their organic status. If animals are sick and alternative treatments (such as allowed herbal remedies) fail, antibiotics, dewormers, or other appropriate synthetic substances should be used to help them.

✔ Treated chickens must be separated from organically raised chickens, and their eggs and meat can't be labeled organic.

✔ **Don't save mixed vaccine for later use — it won't work.** Many poultry vaccines contain live virus, which heat and sunlight quickly inactivate. For example, the virus in Marek's disease vaccine lasts only about two hours after the vaccine is mixed in preparation for use.

✔ **Before you use a vaccine, read the vaccine label and package insert.** Vaccines have expiration dates and withdrawal times as well as directions for preparing and giving the vaccine, which are all listed on the label and package insert.

Giving Medications and Vaccinations

If you do decide to medicate or vaccinate, and you've received the meds or vaccines to give your flock, you need to know how to properly administer them. Several routes are available, and they all have their advantages and challenges.

People with severe cases of *trypanophobia* (fear of needles) may want to skip most of this section, because the surefire ways to get medication and vaccinations into chickens involve needles. Any backyard flock keeper can become adept at the injection techniques that we describe. If the thought of wielding sharp objects around your chickens makes you uncomfortable, we encourage you to find a mentor — a veterinarian, vet technician, or experienced flock keeper, for example — to show you how.

Don't throw needles, stabber tools, syringes, and vaccine vials in the trash or recycling bin, or try to flush them down the toilet. Somebody can get hurt. Here's how to properly dispose of needles and other sharp objects used for medicating or vaccinating chickens:

✔ **Put needles, other sharps, vaccine vials, and syringes in a sharps disposal container immediately after you're done using them.** Your local pharmacy sells FDA-approved sharps containers, or in a pinch, you can use a heavy-duty plastic household container, such as an empty laundry detergent bottle. The container should be leak-proof and have a tight fitting lid. Label the container clearly: "Do not recycle: household sharps."

✔ **Dispose of used sharps containers according to the rules where you live.** Ask your veterinarian or pharmacist if they can take the container and dispose of it for you, or if they know of a local sharps disposal program. If the veterinarian or pharmacist can't help you, call your county or city government agency responsible for trash pickup or public health and ask about the sharps disposal program for your community.

In drinking water

Drinking water is the most common route for giving medications to poultry flocks. Also, some vaccinations are given in drinking water. Here are the pros and cons to using this method:

✔ **Pros:** Medicated drinking water is a practical way to treat several birds or a whole flock at once. It's the least stressful way to medicate a chicken.

✔ **Cons:** Sick birds may not drink enough water to get an adequate dose of the medication. In hot weather, chickens drink more and may overdose themselves.

Each day you provide medicated drinking water to the flock, clean the waterer and mix a fresh batch of medicated solution according to the label directions.

Use nonreactive plastic or ceramic waterers for medicated water, instead of metal. Medicated solutions in metal waterers are a recipe for corrosion or who-knows-what kind of chemical reactions.

By mouth

Although needle-phobic people and people new to flock keeping prefer this method, the oral route is our least favorite method of getting medication into a chicken. Here are the pros and cons for this method:

- ✓ **Pros:** This method doesn't involve needles and their disposal issues.

- ✓ **Cons:** Forcing liquid or pills down a chicken's throat is stressful for you and the chicken. In fact, there's a chance the medication will go down the wrong hole (the windpipe). You also never know whether a good dose went into the chicken or if most of the dose is all over your shirt.

If you must give medication to a chicken by mouth, here are a couple of tips and a warning:

You can mix liquids, crushed tablets, or the powder from opened capsules with a special treat and feed it to an individually-housed sick chicken. Mix the dose with a small amount of food that you know the bird will immediately consume. Mini peanut butter sandwiches, canned corn kernels, rice, cooked sweet potato, or smashed hard-boiled eggs are hits for most birds, even ones who aren't feeling great.

You can slowly administer liquid medications drop by drop into the mouth. To give tablets, you can hold a chicken's beak open with her head extended and toss a pill (or pieces of pills) to the back of the throat. Close the beak and hope for a swallow.

If the chicken starts to struggle as you're giving a medication by mouth, or if she seems to have trouble breathing and medication starts coming out of her nostrils, immediately release the chicken. (Put your hands up and step away from the chicken!) Allow her to clear her own throat.

Eyedrop

Giving vaccinations through eyedrops is a simple method. Some poultry vaccines, including the ILT vaccine, are given as a drop of liquid in a chicken's eye. To administer eyedrops, follow these steps:

1. **Round up the flock and have the birds ready to vaccinate all at one time before you open and mix the vaccine.**

   Having someone there to catch and hold each bird for you makes the job easier.

2. **Mix the vaccine according to the label directions and wash your hands after mixing the vaccine.**

3. **Work quickly to vaccinate all the birds in the group at the same time.**

   Eyedrop vaccine contains live virus that doesn't survive long after the vaccine is mixed. Keep the mixed vaccine cool. Don't save leftover vaccine; it won't work if you save it and use it on another day.

4. **Gently hold the chicken's beak closed with the head tilted to the side.**

5. **Place one drop of vaccine in one eye, as we show in Figure 16-1.**

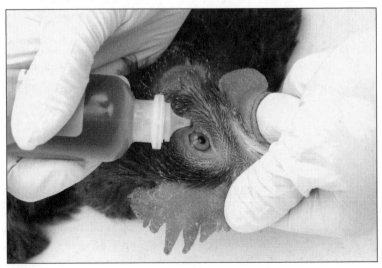

Figure 16-1: Giving an eyedrop vaccine.

Photograph courtesy of Dave Gauthier, PhD

6. **Wait until you see the bird swallow before you release it.**

   It's also okay if the drop goes in the nostril instead of the eye — just wait until the chicken inhales the drop before you let it go.

   A day or two after vaccination, the inoculated eye may look a little sore, but it should pass within a week or so.

Wing web stab

Giving vaccine through a wing web stab isn't as brutal as it sounds. In fact, this method is a quick and easy way to vaccinate poultry. Several poultry vaccines, such as vaccines for fowl pox, avian encephalomyelitis (AE), and fowl cholera, are given by injection into the skin. The web of skin between the upper and lower wing bones is a convenient patch of skin to use on a chicken, because it doesn't seem to be a very sensitive area, and it's easy to find. Here's how to vaccinate a flock of chickens in the wing web:

1. **Ask someone to help you catch and hold the birds.**

   Make sure you also have the vaccine vials and the wing web stabber tool nearby. (The stabber tool should be provided with the vaccine when you purchase it.)

2. **Mix the vaccine according to the instructions provided by the vaccine manufacturer and wash your hands after mixing the vaccine.**

   Keep the stabber and the vaccine vials as clean as possible while you're preparing and giving the vaccine.

3. **Work quickly to vaccinate all the birds in the group at the same time.**

   Vaccine given in the wing web contain live virus that doesn't survive long after you mix it. Keep the mixed vaccine cool. Don't save leftover vaccine; it won't work if you save it to use on another day.

4. **Find the wing web as shown in Figure 16-2.**

   The person holding each bird should spread one wing with the underside facing upward. You may need to pluck a few little feathers in the wing web area to get a clear view of the skin.

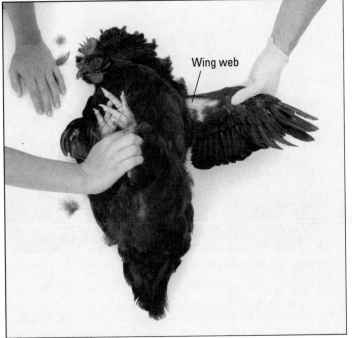

Wing web

Photograph courtesy of Dave Gauthier, PhD

Figure 16-2: Locating the wing web.

5. **Dip the two needles of the stabbing tool into the vaccine liquid.**

6. **Poke the needles *all the way through* the wing web, avoiding bones, muscles, and blood vessels.**

   Don't worry. This step isn't difficult, because there isn't much bone or muscle or many blood vessels in that area, just skin. See Figure 16-3. Stab like you mean it — a confident stab gets the job done faster and easier for you and the bird.

7. **Remove the needles and set the bird down.**

   She'll shake it off and, in 30 seconds or so, appear as if she forgot it ever happened.

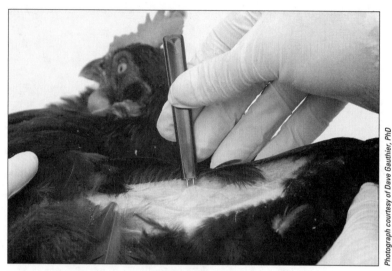

Figure 16-3: Inserting the needle in the wing web.

8. **One week later, check the wing web of each bird for a sign of a successful vaccination, called a *take*.**

You should see two swollen bumps or two scabs in the skin where you gave the vaccine. If you don't see any sign of a reaction in the wing web area, you should revaccinate that bird.

Vaccinate the same wing (right or left) on each bird so you know which side to check later.

Under the skin

You can administer Marek's disease vaccine and some types of medications through a needle inserted subcutaneously (SQ), beneath the skin. Here are some upsides and downsides to using this method:

- ✔ **Pros:** This method is quick, easy, and less stressful than oral medication. You know for certain that the chicken got the dose.

- ✔ **Cons:** The chicken's body slowly absorbs the medication given subcutaneously. Missing the SQ space and injecting into a blood vessel or air sac is possible.

Here's how to give a chick a Marek's disease vaccine subcutaneously:

1. **Start with 1 mL syringes and short needles.**

   One-half to three-quarter inches long and 20- to 22-gauge needles work well. You can get syringes and needles from farm stores, pharmacies, veterinary supply companies, or your veterinarian.

2. **Round up supplies and chicks and have everything ready before you mix the vaccine, because you need to use the mixed vaccine quickly (within two hours).**

   Keep the mixed vaccine cool on an ice pack while you're administering it.

3. **Hold each chick in your nondominant hand with its head pointed toward your other hand.**

   With your thumb and first finger, pinch the skin on the back of the chick's neck just below the head.

4. **Pick up the syringe and needle in your dominant hand and insert the needle into the tent made by the pinched neck skin, close to the head, with the needle pointed toward the chick's body.**

   Figure 16-4 shows how to do so.

5. **Inject the vaccine.**

   If vaccine liquid spills out, you've missed and gone all the way through the skin. It's okay; just try again.

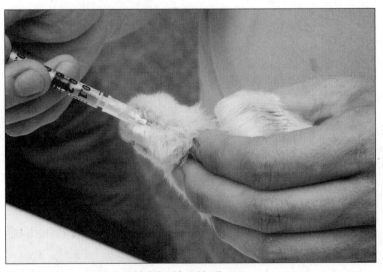

Figure 16-4: Vaccinating a chick for Marek's disease.

Photograph courtesy of Dave Gauthier, PhD

If you need to subcutaneously inject a larger chicken with a medication, you can use a procedure that is similar to the one we describe for the chick. You should have someone help you hold a larger bird while you pick up the skin on the back of the neck with one hand and inject the medication into the tent of skin with the syringe in your other hand. See Figure 16-5 for correct positioning of the needle.

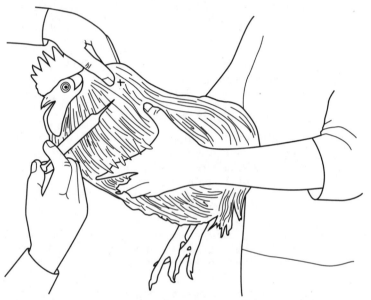

Figure 16-5: A subcutaneous injection for an adult chicken.

In the muscle

The size and thickness of chicken breast muscles make an easy target and a safe area for intramuscular (IM) injection of medications or vaccinations. Here are the pros and cons to this method.

- ✔ **Pros:** The chicken seems to fuss less over an intramuscular (IM) injection than she does over medication by mouth. An IM shot is definitely quicker, easier, and surer for the flock keeper than is the oral medication rodeo.

- ✔ **Cons:** IM injections can be irritating and make a chicken sore.

You almost can't miss. It's easy to give a chicken an IM injection; just follow these steps:

1. **Start with short needles.**

   The best are ½- to ¾-inch, 20- to 22-gauge needles. Your veterinarian can provide you with supplies, or you can purchase syringe and needles from farm stores or mail-order vet supply companies.

2. **Have someone hold the bird for you.**

3. **Feel the *keel* (a ridge of bone down the center of the breast) and feel the wide breast muscles on either side of the keel.**

4. **Insert the needle at a 45-degree angle into the breast muscle an inch to one side of the keel bone, as Figure 16-6 shows.**

5. **Inject all the medication in the syringe before withdrawing the needle.**

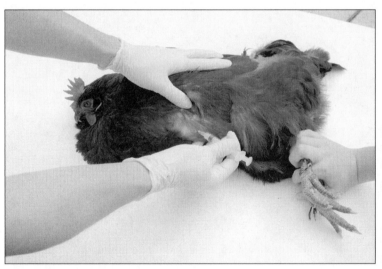

Photograph courtesy of Dave Gauthier, PhD

Figure 16-6: Intramuscular injection in the breast muscle.

Chapter 17

Performing Chicken Maintenance and First-Aid Procedures

In This Chapter

▶ Taking care of your chickens' grooming needs and performing minor maintenance procedures

▶ Assembling a backyard flock first-aid plan

*T*his chapter is a how-to manual of do-it-yourself chicken grooming and repair procedures. We show you how to trim wings, toenails, spurs, and beaks, and we demonstrate placing *peepers* on an aggressive hen who can't get along. In chatting with poultry-fan acquaintances, you may hear about some classic chicken surgeries, such as neutering or dubbing a rooster; we brief you on those procedures in this chapter, but note that a backyard flock keeper rarely, if ever, needs to use those skills.

We also delve into the topic of chicken first aid in this chapter. Isolating a sick or injured chicken and providing supportive care in a hospital cage is probably more helpful than any drug you can give. Backyard flock keepers only need to have a few inexpensive supplies on hand to be prepared to deal with most chicken emergencies.

Giving Your Chicken a Spa Treatment

Chicken pedicures and wing trims aren't just good grooming; they're also preventive health care — for both the chicken and you. For example, long nails and wicked rooster spurs can cause serious damage to flock mates and also to human handlers. These sections point out the important areas for you to take care of with your chicken.

Don't feel like you have to go it alone with any of these procedures, although many flock keepers competently perform them at home on their own birds. If you don't feel comfortable performing any of the procedures in this section, a veterinarian with an interest in chickens or an experienced flock keeper can help you, either by doing the job for you, or showing you how to do it.

Trimming a wing

The main reason to trim a chicken's wing is to prevent the bird from flying out of an uncovered yard. Most chickens are content to stay on their side of the fence, but a few have an urge to wander. Roaming chickens risk becoming a lively but short-lived plaything for a neighborhood dog, or facing the wrath of a homeowner with a soiled patio or vehicle to clean.

Before you assume an escapee hen has wanderlust, examine her social situation. A roaming chicken may be afraid to stay in the pen because of persecution by flock mates. You can trim her wing, but also provide a get-away cage, a straw bale cave, or some other refuge from harassment.

Trimming one wing seems to be more effective than trimming both, because it unbalances the bird as well as reduces lift. Pick a side, any side. The procedure is quick and easy, especially if you have someone to hold the bird for you. Here's how to trim a wing:

1. **Ask the person holding the bird to stretch out one wing and expose the long flight feathers.**

   The longest feathers at the end of the wing are called the *primary flight* feathers or *primaries;* most chickens have ten of them, and these ten feathers are the ones you trim. Find the *coverts,* which are a layer of shorter feathers overlapping the primaries.

2. **Using a sharp pair of scissors, cut each of the ten primaries about an inch below where the coverts end, as shown in Figure 17-1.**

   Avoid trimming any new, emerging tube-shaped pinfeathers, which may bleed if they're cut short.

A wing trim is a temporary measure. When the trimmed chicken molts next (typically once a year in the fall), she'll shed the clipped feathers and grow a full new set of flight-sustaining plumage.

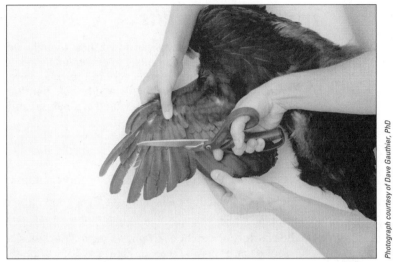

Figure 17-1: You can trim a wing with a pair of scissors.

The trimmed wing should look like the one in Figure 17-2. When the wing is folded, you won't notice the trimmed feathers.

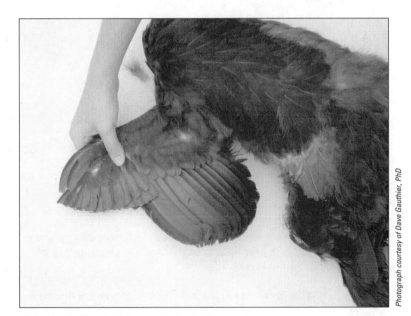

Figure 17-2: What a trimmed wing looks like.

Trimming toenails

Foraging chickens normally wear down their toenails during their scratching activities, but toenails can occasionally become over-grown, especially if a bird spends a lot of time on a wire cage floor. Long toenails can gouge flock mates and human handlers. They can also get snagged and torn off, which is a painful and bloody event.

The right tool for the job depends on the bird's size:

- ✔ Children's nail clippers work well for tiny bantam chickens.

- ✔ Guillotine-style dog nail trimmers are a good choice for your average-size hen.

- ✔ Heavy-duty sheep hoof trimmers make short work of paring stout rooster claws (refer to Figure 17-3).

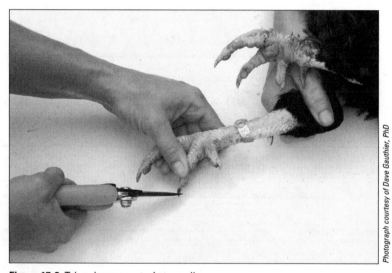

Photograph courtesy of Dave Gauthier, PhD

Figure 17-3: Trimming a rooster's toenails.

Trimmed toenails are still sharp. You can smooth the edges with a nail file or a hand-held rotary tool with a cone-shaped abrasive tip, as shown in Figure 17-4.

Even the most experienced chicken groomers occasionally draw blood while trimming toenails. It's no problem if you do. Just stop the bleeding by dipping the nail into cornstarch, pressing the nail into a bar of soap, using a styptic pencil or powder, or applying pressure with a damp tea bag. After you get it to stop bleeding, you can seal the cut end of the toenail with a dab of instant glue.

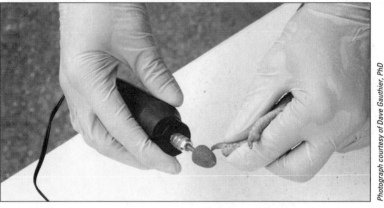

Figure 17-4: You can shape a toenail and smooth the edges.

Trimming rooster spurs

Roosters appear to be very proud of their spurs and know how to use them. However, you may need to take down that pride a notch or two, because a rooster can lacerate the backs of his hens with those glorious leg appendages, and he can hurt people if he attacks to defend his harem. You can use one of two methods to trim your rooster's spurs, which we discuss in these sections.

Uncapping spurs

Uncapping a rooster spur removes the horn-like covering to the bone inside the spur and leaves the spur shorter and more pliable. This procedure works well on mature roosters with long spurs; you usually repeat it annually. It's not painless, but it's quick, and the rooster seems to forget the insult almost immediately. Here's how to uncap a rooster spur:

1. **Ask the person holding the rooster to extend the bird's leg and hold it still for you.**

   With a stout pair of pliers, clamp the spur near its base, as shown in Figure 17-5.

2. **Holding the pliers closed gently but firmly on the spur, rock the handles back and forth slightly until you feel the spur cap loosen.**

   To get this motion right, imagine you're trying to unscrew a bolt with the pliers using gentle back and forth persuasion.

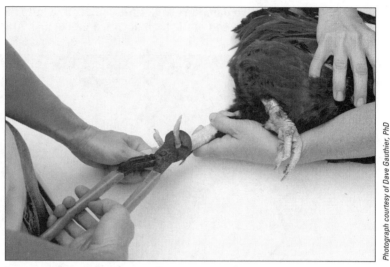

Photograph courtesy of Dave Gauthier, PhD

Figure 17-5: Grasp a rooster's spur near the base to uncap it.

3. **Give a good turn with the pliers, and the cap should come off as you pull the closed pliers away from the leg.**

   The bone underneath the cap is now exposed (see Figure 17-6); it will ooze a little blood, but not much. You can leave it alone and allow the spur stump to air-dry, which it will in a few minutes. You can squeeze a damp tea bag around the spur stump for a minute or two, or you can sprinkle it with some styptic powder.

4. **Repeat the procedure for the spur on the other leg.**

   Give the rooster a break from his ladies for the night (in a separate cage), because they'll be curious about (and peck at) his freshened appearance.

Blunting spurs

Blunting a spur is basically a nail trim, although you're trimming the spurs. Like a nail trim, you must repeat this procedure every few months to keep the spur short. You can cut off approximately the last one-third of a spur's length without encountering a blood vessel. We use sheep hoof trimmers in Figure 17-7, but sharp pruners or a rotary cutting tool also work well. After trimming the spur, shape the tip smooth with a nail file or a hand-held rotary tool with a conical abrasive tip.

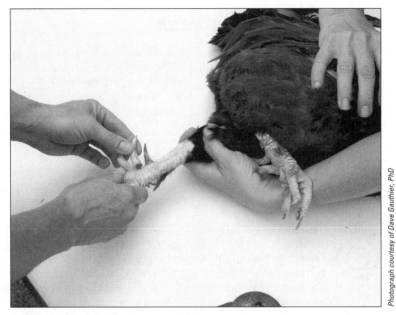

Figure 17-6: An example of an uncapped spur.

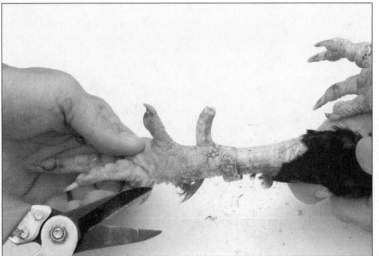

Figure 17-7: You can use sheep hoof trimmers to blunt a spur.

A spur cut too short bleeds profusely. If you use the spur blunting method, be prepared with some form of blood-stopping tool, such as a styptic pencil or powder, and a tube of instant glue to seal it. It will take time and patience to stop the bleeding.

Trimming a beak

Bird beaks and human fingernails are made of the same stuff: *keratin.*
Like human fingernails, a bird's beak grows continuously, and it can
become overgrown, especially if the bird doesn't get a lot of pecking-
in-the-dirt exercise. You may have seen one of your chickens maintaining her beak by filing it side to side on cement or stone.

An overlong beak is prone to splitting, chipping, or other damage,
so trimming it is a good idea. A beak trim is also part of routine
grooming to prepare for a poultry show. Few backyard chickens
need regular beak trimming, but those that are prone to growing
overlong beaks typically need a trim every couple of months.

 Usually, only the tip of the upper beak needs trimming. The trim-
mable portion that lacks blood vessels appears translucent. You
can easily identify these tips on birds with light-colored beaks, but
you may need a bright light, such as an LED flashlight to see the
translucent portion of the tip of dark-colored beaks. Human toenail
clippers work well for trimming bantam chickens' beaks, and sheep
hoof trimmers can tackle larger birds' beaks. After trimming the tip,
as shown in Figure 17-8, shape and smooth the edge with a nail file.

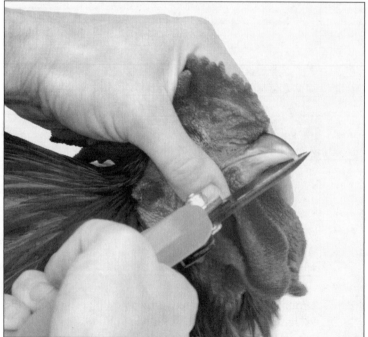

Photograph courtesy of Dave Gauthier, PhD

Figure 17-8: Trimming the tip of a rooster's beak.

A chicken's beak can grow crookedly as a result of incubation temperature errors, injury, malnutrition, or heredity. Severe malformations, such as *crossed beak,* can cause a chicken to be sickly because she can't eat well or preen effectively. Regular beak trimming and reshaping may make a life or death difference for birds with beaks that develop abnormally.

Consult an avian veterinarian for advice and reshaping of a malformed beak, because bird vets commonly treat this condition in a variety of pet birds. Some bird vets are skilled at *rhamphorthotic* techniques (the bird version of orthodontics) to correct a damaged or malformed beak.

Installing peepers

Peepers, also called *blinders* or *chicken spectacles,* are plastic thingies that a chicken wears on her face full-time to partially block her vision and prevent her from bullying her flock mates. Figure 17-9 shows an example of a bespectacled hen. You can use this device as a next-to-last resort for recidivist feather peckers, vent peckers, and chicken cannibals. Backyard chickens can perform all the normal activities of daily living (except pecking each other with accuracy) while wearing peepers, which you can purchase online from poultry supply companies.

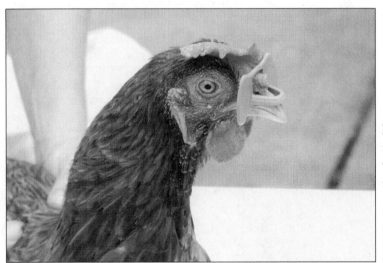

Photograph courtesy of Dave Gauthier, PhD

Figure 17-9: A hen wearing peepers.

You can find several styles of peepers. Some versions require the installation of a nylon or metal pin through the nostrils. Because pin or clip style peepers penetrate and permanently alter the beak (think of it as a pierced nose), some people consider the devices to be inhumane. (In fact, flock keepers in the United Kingdom can't legally use them.) Another style of peepers, which are pinless, grasp but don't completely penetrate the nostrils (sort of like clip-on earrings). Research shows that chickens find them annoying, but most people don't consider them inhumane, especially because the alternative for a cannibalistic hen is execution.

We show you how to install pinless peepers in Figure 17-10. You need a helper to hold the chicken and a pair of snap ring pliers to stretch the peepers open a little. The following steps describe how to do it:

1. **Place the tips of the snap ring pliers in the open space in the center of the peeper device.**

2. **Squeeze the handles of the pliers to stretch out the central opening of the peepers so you can slide the device over the chicken's beak.**

3. **Find the two tabs sticking out from the device and center these tabs over the chicken's nostrils.**

4. **Relax your squeeze on the plier handles to allow the peepers to contract and the tabs to slide into the nostril openings slightly.**

5. **Repeat Steps 1 to 4 if you miss.**

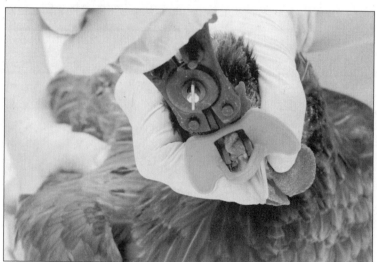

Photograph courtesy of Dave Gauthier, PhD

Figure 17-10: Installing pinless peepers with snap ring pliers.

Don't try this at home: Advanced elective chicken surgery

You're likely to hear about these three elective procedures in poultry circles. None is necessary for backyard flock keeping, and for the chicken's sake, we recommend that you consult a veterinarian or an experienced flock keeper if you're thinking about attempting them at home.

✔ **Debeaking:** *Debeaking* is a permanent alteration of the chicken's pecking apparatus. The most common type of debeaking procedure removes one-third of the upper beak using a hot knife or an infrared light beam. Commercial egg-laying chickens and turkeys are routinely debeaked to prevent feather pecking, vent pecking, and cannibalism. Debeaked chickens can't forage outdoors as effectively as chickens with natural beaks.

✔ **Neutering a rooster:** Also called *caponization,* this antiquated procedure is used to produce meat chickens from slow-growing heritage breed chicken flocks. Just like steers (castrated cattle), neutered male chickens *(capons)* grow bigger at a faster rate and have more tender meat than males that keep their testicles. Unlike cattle anatomy, a male bird's testicles are internal, and bird castration is tricky abdominal surgery. Because broilers can be harvested at a young and tender age, this risky surgical procedure has become obsolete. Caponization doesn't stop a rooster from crowing, after he's learned how to do it (unless he doesn't survive the procedure).

✔ **Removing combs, wattles, and earlobes:** Referred to as *dubbing,* this procedure removes a chicken's comb, wattles, and earlobes, usually with a sharp pair of scissors and without anesthesia. Like ear cropping for show or fighting dogs, dubbing is performed on game breed (gamefowl) roosters for cosmetic or competition purposes — exhibition or cockfighting. A rooster in rare cases is dubbed for medical reasons, particularly to deal with frostbite damage. Because cosmetic dubbing is all about the look and not the chicken's health, a flock keeper interested in dubbing should find an experienced gamefowl stylist as a mentor.

Taking Care of Your Flock: Chicken First Aid

The goal of first aid for a chicken is to provide some relief from suffering caused by illness or injury. First responders don't know at the time when they come to a chicken's aid whether the ultimate outcome is to save a bird's life, restore it to health, stop an injury from worsening, or simply to provide some comfort before the end of life.

Less is better when it comes to first-aid treatments and handling a sick or hurt bird. Stress and pain can tip a sick or injured chicken over the edge of survival. If you decide you must handle a sick or injured bird, perform your treatment quickly and calmly.

Triage a chicken's emergency by addressing the issues in this priority:

- **Life-threatening injuries or illness:** Immediately treat severe bleeding, puncture wounds from predator bites, or collapse from hypothermia or heat exhaustion.

- **Nonlife-threatening injuries or illness that cause severe pain:** Deal with broken bones and deep wounds after you stop the bleeding.

- **Minor injuries or illness:** Give an injured chicken (and yourself) some time to calm down before you treat sore eyes, scrapes, and minor cuts.

Knowing your first-aid philosophy

How you keep your chickens determines how well stocked your backyard flock first-aid kit should be and your philosophy for treating sick or injured birds. Some flock keepers promptly *cull* (kill) a sick or injured bird to relieve suffering, rather than spending effort and expense in a doubtful attempt to return a chicken to a productive life. Others invest great care and expense in the hope of restoring a pet chicken to her active role in the family.

Regardless of how you raise chickens, you should figure out what your philosophy is. No matter what it is, make sure you prepare a chicken first-aid kit with two essentials: a hospital cage in which to assess and isolate a sick or injured bird, and a humane method of euthanasia (see Chapter 18).

We suggest the following items for flock keepers who are inclined to perform some urgent care for chicken emergencies:

- A spare heat lamp and bulb (non-shatterproof) or other heat source to warm a chilled bird (especially chicks)

- An electric fan, mister, or other cooling device to cool an overheated chicken

- An antiseptic solution, such as a dilute Dakin's solution (see the appendix for the recipe) and a 10-mL syringe for flushing wounds

- A pair of forceps (tweezers) for examining wounds and picking out debris, and a pair of scissors for removing bandages

✔ A package of gauze sponges for blotting and cleaning wounds

✔ A method to stop bleeding, such as blood-stop powder, a styptic pencil, cornstarch, or a tea bag

✔ A roll of 1-inch wide adhesive cloth bandaging tape, and a roll of 2-inch wide self-cling bandaging tape for dressing injured feet or wings

✔ A package or bottle of a poultry vitamin and electrolyte preparation to mix with drinking water

✔ A tube of water-based personal lubricant for dealing with a prolapsed vent or suspected egg-bound bird (See Chapter 8)

✔ Your veterinarian's phone number

Treating injuries

The most common backyard chicken injuries are the result of predator attacks, flock-mate aggression, and entanglement in or impalement by objects in the environment, such as broken wire fences or protruding nails. In the following sections we provide a few tips for immediate care of injured chickens.

Stopping bleeding

The bloodiest bird wounds involve injured combs, beaks, toenails, and spurs. Remarkably, lacerations (tears) in chicken skin usually don't bleed much. Applying pressure to an injury with a gauze sponge for a few minutes usually suffices to stop bleeding.

After you get the bleeding under control with pressure, you can sprinkle some blood-stop powder, which is sold at farm stores, on the oozing wound. You can also dab some instant glue on a damaged comb, beak, toenail, or spur to cover and protect the area.

Treating wounds

If a chicken survives an attack by a predator, the next battle to fight is infected bite wounds. A predator's teeth drive wound-festering germs deep into flesh. Cat bites, in particular, are highly likely to become infected. To prevent a life-threatening infection in a traumatized chicken, treat bite wounds and other puncture wounds or skin tears as soon as you discover them.

To treat a wound, you need plenty of wound-flushing solution, such as a dilute Dakin's solution (it's cheap and easy to make; see the recipe in the appendix), a 10-mL syringe, and a pair of forceps (tweezers). Here's what to do:

1. **Wash your hands with soap and water and put on disposable gloves if you have them.**

2. **Wrap the chicken in a towel to calm and restrain her.**

   Wrapping the chicken also soaks up any excess flush solution.

3. **Pluck the feathers from the edges of the wounds to give you a clear view of the area.**

4. **Fill the syringe with the antiseptic solution, and using some pressure on the plunger of the syringe, jet the solution through the wound to flush it.**

   You may need to repeat the flush several times to get the wound clean.

5. **Remove feathers, leaves, and other debris from the wound with the forceps.**

6. **Keep the chicken by herself in a hospital cage until the wound heals.**

7. **Repeat the wound cleaning each day for three to five days.**

8. **Wash your hands with soap and water after treating the bird each time.**

The usefulness of applying topical medicine such as an antibiotic ointment to chicken wounds is doubtful, so we don't recommend it. A bird's own preen gland oil has antibacterial properties and skin conditioners that are just right for bird skin, so allow your injured chicken to preen and take care of the wound herself, rather than slather it with interfering ointment. Your veterinarian can advise you whether giving antibiotics by mouth or by injection is a good idea.

You don't need to stitch up bite wounds and lacerations on chickens. In fact, leave them open because they're usually dirty by the time you find them, and dirty wounds stitched closed are great places for nasty bacteria to flourish. Even a large tear in a chicken's skin will eventually heal if it's left open and the chicken is allowed to take care of it herself by preening around the wound. Consult your veterinarian if you believe a wound should be stitched. (Oh, and did you know that birds are highly resistant to tetanus? They don't need tetanus shots.)

Treating broken bones

A chicken has a *fracture* (a broken bone) if you can see an odd angle to a limb (compared to the other limb), see swelling and red or green bruising, and feel a grinding sensation as you run your fingers over the swollen spot.

However, most limping chickens and most chickens with a drooping wing *don't* have a broken bone. Limping and droopy wings are very common signs of nerve damage due to incurable Marek's disease (see Chapter 12).

A *closed* fracture is a break in a bone that doesn't tear the surrounding skin open; an *open* fracture describes a break where the bone can be seen through an open wound in the skin. In Table 17-1, you can see an important difference between the treatment and prognosis for closed versus open fractures in chickens. Open fractures in chicken limbs are likely to become infected and heal poorly, if at all, without medical and surgical intervention. Because of the pain and peril associated with open fractures in chicken limbs, we recommend that you consult a veterinarian about treatment, or if that's not an option, euthanize the bird to relieve suffering.

Table 17-1 Managing Backyard Chicken Limb Fractures

Location	Type of Fracture	Prognosis	Management
Wing	Closed	Good	Apply a figure-8 bandage and confine for 2 to 3 weeks
Wing	Open	Fair to poor	Consult a veterinarian or euthanize
Leg	Open or closed	Poor	Consult a veterinarian or euthanize
Toe	Closed	Good	Confine for 2 to 3 weeks
Toe	Open	Fair	Bandage and confine for 2 to 3 weeks

Because chickens don't have to make a living by flying, most closed wing fractures aren't too serious and don't need to be perfectly realigned for the bird to do well. Flock keepers can manage most wing fractures by bandaging the wing and confining the chicken to a hospital cage for two to three weeks.

A figure-8 bandage is a simple way to support and immobilize an injured wing. You need a roll of 2-inch self-cling bandage tape (found in the horse supply section of farm stores) and someone to hold the bird for you. Here's how to wrap the bandage:

1. **Unwrap and re-roll the whole roll of bandage tape.**

   Doing so loosens the tape and helps prevent you from wrapping the bandage too tightly.

2. **Hold the injured wing in the normal closed (flexed) position.**

3. **Wrap the tape in a figure-8 pattern around the injured wing, as shown in Figure 17-11.**

   You can repeat the pattern with a couple of layers of wrap.

4. **Continue the wrap over the bird's back and around the body.**

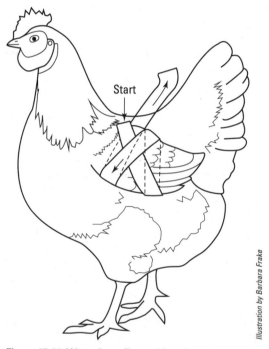

Start

Illustration by Barbara Frake

Figure 17-11: Wrapping a figure-8 bandage to support an injured wing.

Leave the uninjured wing out of the body wrap. The bandage should go underneath the bird at the middle of the keel, and then up and over the injured wing, holding it against the body. Go around the body with the wrap one more time.

The body wrap should be tight enough to prevent the wing from moving but not tight enough to restrict breathing. Make sure you can fit two fingers in the gap between the injured wing and the body.

Leg fractures in chickens are a different story from wing fractures; they're rarely a successful do-it-yourself project. A poorly applied splint can do more harm than good, and many avian leg fractures are more successfully treated with surgery rather than splinting. In addition to the challenge of immobilizing the broken leg, a chicken's uninjured leg is likely to develop the painful condition of *bumblefoot* (see Chapter 14) as a consequence of taking all the strain for several weeks. For these reasons, we suggest you seek advice from your veterinarian if you want to try to heal a chicken with a broken leg.

Giving some TLC for sick or injured chickens

A clean, comfortable, and well-fed bird has amazing recuperative powers, so a sick or injured chicken may benefit more from your supportive nursing care than any drugs you can give. Here's how to help:

- ✔ **Isolate the chickens.** Chickens take advantage of a down-and-out flock mate to express their dominance, and they relentlessly investigate a flock mate's wounds and make the injury worse. (The other hens think, "Oooh, pretty — a shiny red spot!") Separate a sick or injured chicken from the rest of the flock as soon as you discover the problem and keep her in a cage by herself. A large pet carrier works well as a hospital cage. The hospital cage should be placed in an enclosed, but well-ventilated area where no other animals are kept, such as a garage or shed.

- ✔ **The hospital cage should be warm, clean, and comfortable by the chicken's standards.** For chickens more than a month old, find a way to keep the chicken's environment at a stable 80 to 85 degrees Fahrenheit (27 to 29 degrees Celsius). For chicks 4 weeks old or less, maintain room temperature at 90 to 95 degrees F (32 to 35 degrees C). Use non-slip bedding, such as synthetic turf, terrycloth towels, or wood shavings, and keep the cage scrupulously clean, removing droppings promptly. If the bird is accustomed to roosting at night, provide a low, comfortable perch for sleeping.

- ✔ **Use light therapy.** To encourage a sick bird to eat and drink, leave a light on around the clock. To stop a hen with a reproductive tract problem from producing eggs, keep her in the dark for 16 hours a day.

- ✔ **Make it easy for a sick bird to get adequate nutrition.** Chickens are hungriest during the morning, so focus on feeding your sick chicken a good meal at that time. Pelleted feed is the easiest form of commercial diet for adult chickens to consume; crumbles are easiest for chicks. The complete commercial diet can be top-dressed with favorite treats to entice a chicken with a poor appetite. Mashed hard-boiled egg (shell and all), mealworms, pumpkin, yogurt, peanut butter sandwiches, and chopped kale or other greens are examples of nutrient-dense foods that most chickens eagerly consume.

✔ **Stressed, sick, and injured chickens benefit from vitamin supplementation.** Supplemental antioxidant vitamins, particularly vitamins A, C, and E, support chickens' immune systems, aid healing, and help birds cope with stress. You can find poultry vitamin and electrolyte supplements at feed stores or poultry-supply companies to mix with drinking water. Prepare the solution as directed on the label and offer it as the only source of drinking water for the isolated bird.

Some livestock vitamin and electrolyte supplements don't contain vitamin C (ascorbic acid). If that's the type of supplement you have, you can crush a 1000-mg vitamin C tablet and add that to the drinking water along with the supplement.

Chapter 18

Euthanizing a Chicken and Disposing of the Remains

In This Chapter

▶ Deciding to treat or euthanize a sick or injured chicken

▶ Weighing the pros and cons of euthanasia methods

▶ Composting dead birds and other disposal options

*E*uthanasia means a "good death," and our goal in this chapter is to explain this difficult topic. To make that final decision to end a chicken's life and then to act on it is never easy, but knowing how to euthanize a chicken is an important responsibility of every backyard flock keeper. We support you in your decision to close the chicken repair manual and humanely kill a sick or injured chicken.

Three of the four methods we describe are do-it-yourself techniques, performed at home by flock keepers with their own hands. Therefore, this chapter contains descriptions of euthanasia procedures that are detailed and straightforward, which may make some readers uncomfortable.

Depending on where you live, you have several choices for taking care of chicken remains. Factoring into your choice of method for disposing of a dead bird are your community's rules, practicality, and ever-present scavengers. In this chapter, we also compile the main options for backyard flock carcass disposal.

Making the Decision

Weigh your decision whether to treat or to euthanize a sick or injured chicken by asking yourself these questions:

✔ Is the chicken in severe pain or distress?

✔ Is the chicken unlikely to recover?

✔ Is the chicken likely to transmit disease to other birds?

✔ Does the chicken have a disease that poses a risk to human health?

✔ Is treatment unlikely to be successful?

✔ Is the cost of treatment prohibitive?

✔ Will treating the chicken with appropriate medications make its eggs or meat unsafe for human consumption?

If you answered "yes" to any of these questions, euthanasia, rather than treatment, may be justified.

Don't delay your decision to end suffering because of squeamishness or hope for death to occur naturally. Ask someone to help you if you don't feel up to it. We've not yet met a flock keeper who regretted euthanizing a chicken, but we have met some who said, "I wish I hadn't let that chicken suffer so long."

Identifying Humane Methods of Euthanasia

Several methods are available to flock keepers to humanely euthanize backyard chickens. The goal is to kill a chicken as nearly instantaneously as possible with minimal pain and distress for the bird and low risk of harm to people. In Table 18-1, we list accepted methods of poultry euthanasia that are practical in backyard settings and that you or your veterinarian can safely perform.

We make the distinction between euthanasia as an act of mercy for a sick or injured chicken and slaughter of a healthy chicken for food, although some of the methods in Table 18-1 can be used for either euthanasia or slaughter.

Never slaughter a sick chicken for human consumption. A sick chicken isn't safe for people to eat. Slaughter only healthy birds for food.

Table 18-1 Euthanasia Methods for Backyard Chickens

Method	Skill Required	Cost	Limitations	Slaughter for Food
Injection of euthanasia solution	High	High	Solution available only to licensed vets; carcass disposal challenges	No
Cervical dislocation	Moderate	Low	Physically tiring; roosters and larger, older birds are more difficult	Yes, if followed by *exsanguination* (cutting the throat)
CO_2 chamber	Low	Moderate to high	Cost of tank and regulator; tank may freeze up	Yes, if followed by exsanguination
Exsanguination or decapitation	Moderate	Low	Bird should be stunned first; very bloody	Yes

Being prepared and considering bystanders

Almost any method of chicken euthanasia, even when it's delivered swiftly and competently, involves involuntary, unconscious movements by the chicken at the time of death. Be prepared for it.

Dying chickens may exhibit these actions:

- ✔ Flap their wings and kick their legs
- ✔ Gasp
- ✔ Vocalize
- ✔ Appear to contain an incredible amount of blood, if exsanguination or decapitation is used

Reflexive movements and sounds don't indicate awareness or pain sensation.

Consider bystanders who may witness euthanasia or slaughter of a chicken. Choose a private location to carry it out so no one unwittingly sees your activities. If you choose to have witnesses to the process, warn them ahead of time about what you'll do and what they're likely to see.

Injecting a euthanasia solution

A veterinary euthanasia solution containing an anesthetic drug is given by injection into a wing, neck, leg vein, or the abdominal cavity.

- ✔ **Pros:** The injected solution causes rapid unconsciousness and anesthesia before death. When skillfully performed, this method is probably the least painful of the methods we describe.

- ✔ **Cons:** Intravenous injection requires skill; a vein can be difficult to find in very sick birds. Afterwards, the carcass is toxic. Euthanasia by injection may be expensive, relative to the monetary value of the chicken.

Laws restrict the purchase and use of veterinary euthanasia solutions to licensed veterinarians or trained personnel under the supervision of a licensed veterinarian, so this method is obviously not a do-it-yourself option for most backyard flock keepers. If you want to do this method, you transport a sick or injured chicken to your veterinarian's office for the injection, unless your vet makes farm calls.

Your veterinarian may not always be available for emergency euthanasia of an injured chicken, so you should consider a backup plan.

The tissues of the euthanized chicken are full of the anesthetic drug. Pets or scavengers that eat the carcass can be poisoned, possibly fatally. To prevent accidents, ask your veterinarian to dispose of the carcass for you. If you must dispose of the euthanized chicken at home, bury the carcass deeply — cover it with at least two feet of soil — to prevent animals from digging up and eating the remains.

Performing cervical dislocation

Breaking a chicken's neck near the base of the skull (called *cervical dislocation*) damages the lower part of the brain, causing rapid unconsciousness and death. To be humane, dislocation of the neck must separate the brain from both the spinal cord and the arteries that carry blood to the brain.

 ✔ **Pros:** In skilled hands, cervical dislocation causes instant unconsciousness. The method is low cost and requires either just your hands or simple tools, depending on how you do it.

 ✔ **Cons:** Cervical dislocation requires some training, skill, and strength to perform quickly and properly. The method is physically tiring, so it isn't a good option if you need to euthanize more than just one or two birds.

Find an experienced person to show you how to perform this procedure. Practice on a dead chicken to gauge how much force you need to use, before you attempt this for the first time on your own.

Breaking a chick's neck

A young chick's neck can be broken by pinching the neck firmly at the base of the skull between the thumb and index finger. Alternatively, use the inside of the non-cutting angle of a pair of scissors to pinch the neck, as shown in Figure 18-1.

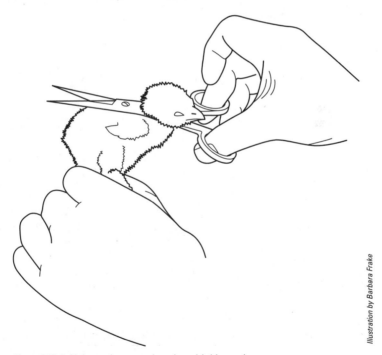

Illustration by Barbara Frake

Figure 18-1: Using scissors to break a chick's neck.

Breaking a hen's neck

To break a hen's or a growing chicken's neck, you use the manual method (refer to Figure 18-2). You can follow these steps:

1. **Hold the bird's legs in one hand against your hip, with the bird's back facing you.**

2. **Grasp the back of the bird's head between the thumb and index finger of your other hand.**

3. **Smoothly and rapidly extend your arm holding the bird's head to stretch the neck.**

4. **At the same time as you stretch the neck, flex your wrist to roll the head backwards.**

   Stretching the neck and pulling the head backwards simultaneously separates the skull from the neck bones with a distinct popping feeling. When this is done properly, the spinal cord breaks, killing the bird instantly.

   You can feel the separation between the skull and the neck bones through the skin of the neck.

5. **To be absolutely certain of death, or to slaughter a chicken for food with this method, cut the throat to allow the chicken to bleed out.**

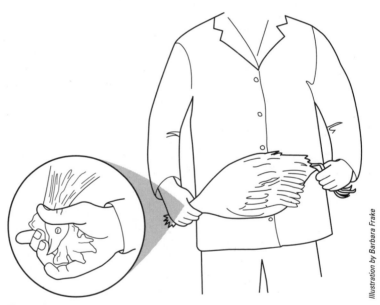

Illustration by Barbara Frake

Figure 18-2: Using your hands to break a hen's neck.

Breaking a rooster's neck

Roosters have powerful neck muscles, so you need a strong person to dislocate a rooster's neck quickly and humanely with hands alone. Using *Burdizzo forceps* is an option for mechanical cervical dislocation of roosters or giant breed chickens. Burdizzo forceps (also known as a Burdizzo clamp or *emasculatome*) are used primarily to castrate cattle. You can purchase the tool from veterinary supply companies.

The procedure is much easier with two people:

1. **One person holds the chicken by the body; the other applies the Burdizzo forceps to the chicken's neck, just below the head, and quickly closes the jaws as far as they will go (as shown in Figure 18-3).**

2. **Leave the tool clamped until reflex movements stop.**

3. **To be absolutely certain of death, or to slaughter the chicken for food, cut the throat to allow the chicken to bleed out.**

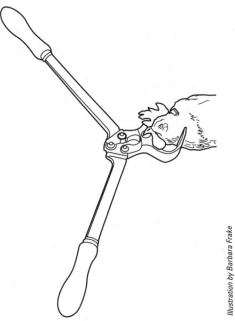

Illustration by Barbara Frake

Figure 18-3: Using Burdizzo forceps to break a large chicken's neck.

Creating a CO_2 chamber

Chickens can be euthanized with carbon dioxide (CO_2) gas in a closed chamber. Breathing the gas at a high enough concentration (50 percent or higher) causes anesthesia and death within two to five minutes.

✔ **Pros:** CO_2 gas produces rapid unconsciousness. It's relatively safe for the operator and bystanders, available almost everywhere, and inexpensive. No blood is spilled, so this method is preferred for euthanizing chickens suspected of having infectious diseases.

✔ **Cons:** Like every other euthanasia method, this one isn't completely pain-free. Breathing CO_2 gas is irritating and causes respiratory distress (gasping for air), albeit briefly.

To make a CO_2 chamber, you need a clear plastic storage box with a lid that latches securely closed (but not airtight), a CO_2 gas cylinder with a regulator, a short length of hose, and a couple of connectors to hook up one end of the hose to the side of the chamber and the other end to the regulator. The box should be big enough for one chicken to stand upright and turn around, and no bigger. See Figure 18-4 for a photo of a CO_2 chamber set up for euthanizing one bird at a time.

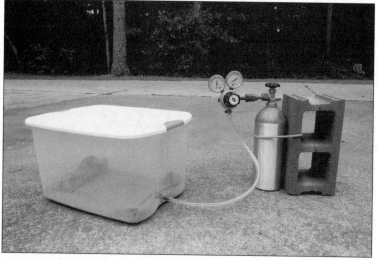

Photograph courtesy of Dave Gauthier, PhD

Figure 18-4: A CO_2 chamber with a gas cylinder.

You can purchase a carbon dioxide cylinder and a regulator from beer-making supply stores or welding supply companies. A five-pound cylinder provides plenty of gas for euthanizing one or a few birds.

To use a CO_2 chamber, follow these steps:

1. **Use the chamber outside, not indoors, and place it on the ground, not up on a table or other surface.** Secure the gas cylinder upright so it can't tip over accidentally.

2. **Place the chicken in the box, latch the lid, and open the cylinder valve slowly to introduce the gas into the chamber.**

Carbon dioxide gas is heavier than air, so the gas fills the chamber from the bottom up, pushing the air out of the small gaps in the lid. (That's why you don't want an airtight box; you want the air to escape out of the top of the chamber.)

After about a minute or two of breathing the gas, the chicken will fall asleep.

3. **Allow the gas to run for two or three more minutes before closing the valve.**

4. **Leave the bird in the box for at least ten minutes to be certain of death.**

You can also use CO_2 gas to stun a chicken for slaughter by exsanguination or decapitation.

You can also use dry ice, instead of a compressed gas cylinder, as the source of CO_2 for the chamber. You can purchase dry ice at many grocery stores, hardware stores, or gas stations. A four- to five-pound (about 2 kg) block of dry ice can easily produce enough gas to euthanize one to five chickens. Get a spare block to hold in reserve, just in case more gas is needed.

Don't put the dry ice in the chamber with the chicken. Make sure you put the dry ice in a separate container so that the chicken can't have direct contact with the freezing substance, which is painful. Don't handle dry ice with your bare hands.

Figure 18-5 shows a set up for a CO_2 chamber with dry ice. Elevate the box containing the dry ice, as shown in the photo, so that heavier-than-air CO_2 vapor rapidly flows down the hose into the chamber holding the chicken. Pour 2 to 3 cups (about ½ liter) of warm water into the box containing the dry ice; doing so causes the solid CO_2 to vaporize more quickly. Make sure the water you add to the box doesn't enter the hose.

Using exsanguination or decapitation

Cutting a chicken's throat to sever the jugular veins and carotid arteries causes the bird to die from blood loss *(exsanguination)*. Full decapitation causes a rapid drop in blood pressure and unconsciousness. Exsanguination and decapitation are considered humane methods of poultry euthanasia or slaughter only if the bird is anesthetized or stunned first. Cervical dislocation, CO_2 gas, or a blow to the head can be used to stun a bird prior to cutting the throat or decapitation.

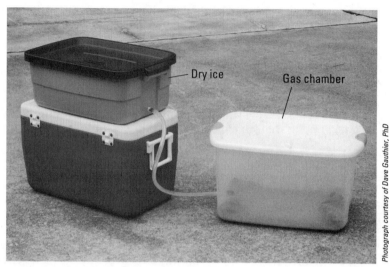

Figure 18-5: A CO_2 chamber with dry ice.

- ✓ **Pros:** Minimal equipment is needed (a sharp knife or a hatchet and chopping block); this is a low-cost method.

- ✓ **Cons:** A surprising amount of skill — both strength and aim — is required for swift, competent decapitation or throat cutting. This method is very bloody, and it's not recommended for euthanizing birds with infectious diseases, because blood can contaminate a wide area.

Considering Disposal Options

Improper disposal of chicken carcasses threatens the health of the rest of your flock, attracts pests, and pollutes soil or water (not to mention creating a horrible odor). In many communities, traditional practices of backyard burning or burial are no longer allowed because of concerns about environmental contamination and risks to human health. Depending on where you live, burial, composting, or putting a carcass in the trash may be legal means for disposing of chicken remains. Make sure you check your community's rules to know your options. Contact your local solid-waste management agency which, in the United States, is usually part of your county's government.

Burial

Where backyard burial is allowed, burying a chicken carcass is practical for most backyard flock keepers. Keep animals from digging up the grave by burying the carcass at least two feet deep, and place wire mesh, bricks, or stones on top of the site. Sprinkling powdered lime on top of the carcass is a traditional custom, but it's not necessary; lime doesn't reliably hasten decomposition or inactivate infectious diseases.

At certain times of the year, you may not be able to dig a hole in frozen soil or hard clay. You can double-bag and freeze a carcass until the ground softens.

Don't bury a carcass near a septic tank, well, or body of water because products from decomposition of the carcass can contaminate nearby groundwater.

Composting

Composting chicken carcasses, when done properly, has several advantages. A properly constructed compost bin or pile

- Doesn't smell bad

- Heats up to 130–150 degrees Fahrenheit (54–65 degrees Celsius) for several days, which inactivates many infectious organisms

- Produces a useable end product — rich, organic compost for your garden or lawn.

Here are basic steps to successfully composting chicken carcasses:

1. **Select a suitable site.**

   Choose a place that has a gentle slope, is out of sight and downwind from neighbors, and is away from drinking-water supplies. Avoid wet locations, such as low areas, under roof gutters, or near drains. Use a compost bin with a scavenger-proof lid, or place wire mesh over the pile to prevent animals from disturbing it.

2. **Gather compost material.**

   A good compost pile contains the right balance of carbon-rich organic materials, nitrogen-rich organic materials, and water. Carbon-rich organic materials are known as *greens,* and nitrogen-rich organic materials are known as *browns.* You need greens, browns, and a water source to build your carcass compost pile. Following are common green sources and brown sources that you probably have access to:

   - **Greens:** Animal manure from coops, stables, or barns; grass clippings; kitchen scraps

   - **Browns:** Straw, hay, wood shavings, sawdust, shredded paper

3. Layer the compost materials.

Twelve inches of greens form the bottom layer of the pile, topped with an inch or two of browns. Chicken carcasses, one bird deep, form the next layer. See Figure 18-6 for the layering scheme. You can repeat the layers three to four times if necessary. Make sure the birds are covered on all sides by at least six inches of compost material, and sprinkle each layer with a little water. Finally, cover the top of the pile with a layer of compost material at least 12 inches thick. Leave this layer dry.

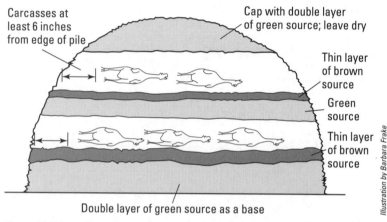

Figure 18-6: Layering a compost pile is an easy process.

4. Wait three weeks and then turn the pile.

Stir the pile by turning it over with a pitchfork or shovel. After turning, let the pile sit and cure for at least three months before using it in the garden or yard.

 For the finer points on the art of composting, refer to other texts on the subject, such as *Composting For Dummies* by Cathy Cromell and the National Gardening Association (John Wiley & Sons, Inc.).

Off-site options

You may be able to put a chicken carcass in the trash or take it to a landfill. Some landfills accept dead animals; check with your household-solid-waste management agency about their policy. If this option is feasible, double-bag the carcass to prevent feathers or fluids from escaping and keep the bag in a scavenger-proof trash receptacle until you can take it to the landfill.

Veterinary clinics, veterinary diagnostic laboratories, and pet cemeteries can also dispose of animal remains for you, for a fee.

Part V
The Chicken/Human Interface

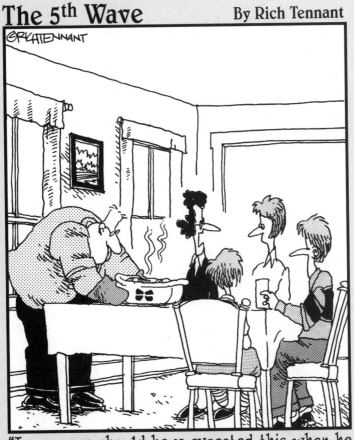

The 5th Wave   By Rich Tennant

@RICHTENNANT

"I guess we should have expected this when he named the chicken, 'Cordon Bleu.'"

In this part...

In this part we describe diseases that chickens and humans can share. We don't want to alarm you, just inform and prevent. Really, few diseases affect both people and chickens, and for most healthy people, the maladies aren't serious. In this part, you can find common-sense advice so you can safely enjoy eggs and meat produced by your flock.

Chapter 19

Can You Get That from a Chicken?

*S*upporters of backyard chickens eagerly point out many benefits that feathered friends provide to flock keepers and their communities. Meanwhile, opponents and regulators of backyard chickens grumble over perceived negative impacts to public health and the community. Along with the usual noise and odor nuisance arguments, critics also cite human health risks. Do they have a point?

Public health practitioners generally agree that raising chickens in backyards isn't riskier than owning a conventional companion animal like a dog or a cat. Very few infectious diseases of chickens are easily transmissible to people, and they usually aren't serious. In this chapter, we describe those chicken-transmitted infections, even the rare ones, and provide common-sense tips on reducing the risk to you, your family, and your neighbors.

Eyeing Two Bacterial Infections You Can Get from Chickens

Health surveys suggest that many cases of diarrheal illness in people around the world are caused by two bacterial infections: *campylobacteriosis* (about 400 million cases each year, worldwide) and *salmonellosis* (about 100 million cases each year, worldwide). If you blame "the runs" on something you ate, chances are you're right, but in a small proportion of cases, your backyard chicken may be the source of the trouble as we discuss in the following list.

- ✔ **Infections in chickens:** Chickens can carry *Campylobacter* and/or *Salmonella* bacteria in their digestive systems, usually without showing any signs of illness. Infected birds pass the bacteria in their droppings, which contaminate the flock's environment and spread the infection to people and other animals that have had contact with the droppings. A few of the thousands of different strains of *Salmonella* can even be passed by an infected hen in her eggs.

  Some surveys have found *Campylobacter* bacteria infecting 90 to 100 percent of sampled flocks. Other research has shown that free-range and organic flocks are just as likely if not more likely than conventional chicken farms to harbor the bacteria. Furthermore, *Salmonella* bacteria are often where flocks are, although less commonly than *Campylobacter*.

  Not much research has been done to find out how often U.S. backyard flocks harbor *Campylobacter* or *Salmonella,* but it's a good bet that at least a small proportion of these flocks has one or both organisms.

- ✔ **Infections in people:** People who catch campylobacteriosis or salmonellosis mainly get it from eating meat that hasn't been cooked thoroughly. Less commonly, the diseases can spread from person to person, or, in about one out of ten cases, from a live animal to a person. Both *Campylobacter* and *Salmonella* bacteria are transmitted by the *fecal-oral route,* which is a nice way of saying that you have to get poop in your mouth in order to catch the disease.

  Poultry are an important source of *Salmonella* and *Campylobacter* bacteria that infect people. In most cases, people contract these bacterial infections through eating contaminated food, particularly chicken meat. A less common way people can get infected is through handling chickens.

  Salmonellosis and campylobacteriosis are nuisances for healthy adult people, causing nausea, vomiting, abdominal cramps, and diarrhea, but they're rarely life-threatening. However, these infections can be serious, possibly fatal, for babies, elderly people, and people with impaired immune systems.

  Don't panic! You can avoid the runs, or worse, with common sense precautions. Read on to find out how you can protect yourself and your family.

Itching at Minor Irritations You Can Get from Chickens

Although itchy skin and irritated eyes are physically uncomfortable, emotionally distressing, and cosmetically unappealing, the chicken-associated maladies in these sections aren't serious human health threats.

Bird mite bites

People can become accidental, temporary hosts for mites that infest chickens and other birds. Mite bites can drive a person crazy; they're intensely itchy, more so at night. The chicken mite, *Dermanyssus gallinae,* which lives near bird nests and comes out at night to feed, is the most common cause of bird mite skin irritations on people. Physicians, even skin specialists, often miss this diagnosis for itchy patients, because the condition is fairly uncommon, and the tiny mites are difficult to spot.

 Check the attic as well as your chickens if you suspect you're being bitten by bird mites. Wild birds nesting in the eaves or attic of a house can also be the source of bird mites. Pestered people can use permethrin shampoo to rid themselves of bird mites, and antihistamines help with the intense itch that can keep a person awake at night. Call an exterminator to discuss treating the house or coop. See Chapter 13 for advice on treating birds for mite infestations.

Wandering lice

Bird lice feed on feathers and feather dander. They're very dependent on their bird hosts, and can live for only a few days if they find themselves birdless and alone in the cold world. If you handle a lousy bird, the pests will crawl on you, but it doesn't take long for hitchhiking bird lice to discover that you are a featherless desert, and leave (in disappointment and disgust, we imagine).

 Poultry farm workers who must handle lousy birds can apply two-sided sticky tape or smear petroleum jelly around their forearms, to prevent the lice from venturing any farther than their arms. If you find yourself temporarily crawling with bird lice, a nice sudsy bath or long hot shower will hasten their departure.

Newcastle disease

Newcastle disease virus infects chickens and many other types of birds. Depending on the virus strain, Newcastle disease in chickens can range from mild respiratory illness and a drop in egg production, to severe nervous system disorders and sudden death (refer to Chapter 12 for more information). Most commercial chicken flocks are vaccinated against Newcastle disease with a live, mild strain of the virus.

People who have contact with Newcastle disease virus, for example, through handling infected birds or giving vaccinations containing live Newcastle disease virus, can become infected. Newcastle disease virus infection in people causes *conjunctivitis* (pink eye), which is an inflammation of the whites of the eyes and the linings of the eyelids. Irritated, blood-shot eyes are uncomfortable and ugly, but not serious, and the infection goes away in five to ten days.

Ringworm

The fungus that causes ringworm *(favus)* in chickens, called *Microsporum gallinae,* can infect the skin or nails of people, though it rarely does. Serious infections with chicken ringworm fungus have been reported to occur in people with immune systems weakened by HIV infection or diabetes.

Treatment for ringworm affecting healthy people is the same whether the fungus originally came from another person, a pet cat, a chicken, or somewhere else. Over-the-counter antifungal medications usually do the trick.

Catching ringworm from a chicken is very rare. If you get ringworm, we suggest you look elsewhere for the source of a ringworm infection.

Naming What You Can Get from Cleaning Chicken Coops

Histoplasmosis and farmer's lung are two human diseases that we can't pin directly on chickens, but people who stir up dust in chicken houses or clean out backyard coops run a higher risk of coming down with them than do people who have nothing to do with birds. These sections explain the possible connection between cleaning coops and these diseases.

Histoplasmosis

Histoplasma capsulatum, the fungus that causes histoplasmosis, lives in the ground, and it particularly likes to live in dirt around old homes, chicken houses, dog kennels, or underneath wild bird roosts. It grows well in caves and can infect people who climb around in them, giving the disease its common name, *caver's disease.* In the United States, the fungus is common in the Ohio River and Mississippi River valleys, and most people who live in those areas have been exposed to the fungus at some point in their lives without ever getting sick from it.

A healthy person probably has to inhale a massive dose of fungal spores in order to come down with histoplasmosis, but people with weak immune systems can more easily become seriously ill if they're exposed to the fungus. If symptoms occur, they usually appear within three days to two weeks of exposure to places where the fungus lives. The signs are similar to the signs of pneumonia, including coughing, fever, and chest pains. Mild cases of histoplasmosis in healthy people usually go away within a month without treatment. More serious cases require months of therapy with strong antifungal medications.

Although the fungus that causes histoplasmosis doesn't live in chickens or in fresh chicken droppings, people with weak immune systems should avoid areas with ancient piles of bird or bat droppings. For people who are taking immunosuppressive medications or who have a debilitating illness, demolishing an old chicken coop isn't just a dirty job, it's potentially dangerous.

To lower your chances of contracting the fungal infection, spray down dusty surfaces with a hose before you start to clean. Don't dry sweep a dusty chicken coop — you may create a cloud of airborne fungal spores. Forget about disinfecting dirt; no chemical will reliably eradicate the fungus from soil.

Farmer's lung

Farmer's lung, also called *hypersensitivity pneumonitis,* is an allergy to inhaled dust from feathers, bird droppings, or moldy stuff, such as hay, straw, or grain. The first exposure for sensitive people creates the allergy, and then every exposure after that triggers an allergic reaction, adding up over time to permanent scarring of the lungs.

Severity of the symptoms of farmer's lung depends on how sensitive the person is and how much dust he or she is exposed to. An attack develops four to eight hours after the dust is inhaled, and can vary from mild flu-like symptoms to coughing up blood and extreme breathing difficulties. The attack usually subsides after 12 hours, but the symptoms of a severe bout can linger many weeks.

You can't find out in advance if you're likely to develop an allergy to dusts generated by birds, but the risk of developing farmer's lung is small, even for people who frequently work in dusty environments.

Contact your doctor if you experience a sudden illness with a cough a few hours after cleaning out a chicken coop or doing another type of dusty job. You can control, but not cure, farmer's lung by avoiding the type of dust that triggers your allergy.

Considering Rare Diseases You Can Get from Chickens

You'd be really unlucky to get one of the rare diseases that we list in this section, but because people are intrigued by the unusual, and fascinated by the freakish, we briefly cover these weird chicken-borne diseases. If we can put your mind at ease that your chicken isn't "Typhoid Henny," or start some unusual dinner table discussions, we're happy to do so. Here is a brief overview of these rare diseases:

- **Bird flu:** Birds are natural hosts for avian influenza viruses, which are closely related to the influenza viruses that are found in humans, horses, pigs, and dogs. Ordinarily, the influenza viruses that are found in each species infect only that species, but sometimes an influenza virus can "jump" from one species to another.

  A deadly version of avian influenza virus called H5N1 has been jumping from birds to people in Asia since 2003. Since then, the H5N1 virus has spread into domesticated poultry and wild birds, and occasionally infected humans in parts of Europe, the Middle East, the Pacific, and Africa. This species-jumping virus hasn't died out yet, however, and public health officials are still keeping an anxious eye on it.

  Almost all cases of human H5N1 infections have been in people who had close contact with infected birds, and most infected people developed severe illness. The mortality rate for people diagnosed with this infection is very scary — two out of every five people known to have the disease have died. So far, fortunately, the spread of H5N1 person to person has been very rare, and this particular strain of avian influenza virus hasn't been found in domesticated poultry in the United States.

- **Erysipeloid:** *Erysipelothrix* bacteria cause disease in many different species, including birds, pigs, and people. The disease in birds and pigs is called *erysipelas;* in people, it's *erysipeloid.* The signs of erysipelas in chickens are dramatic; birds in good condition die suddenly.

This disease is one good reason to wear gloves when handling sick or dead poultry. The infection usually starts at the site of a wound on the person's hand or arm (such as a scratch from a chicken toenail), causing painful swelling, skin discoloration, and blisters. Often, erysipeloid goes away on its own in two to four weeks, and taking penicillin or another antibiotic can speed up recovery. Rarely, the infection can spread to other parts of the body and cause serious illness.

✔ **Avian tuberculosis:** All bird species, including chickens, are susceptible to infection with the bacteria that cause avian tuberculosis. Avian TB causes older chickens (typically older than 2 years) to slowly waste away. The disease, caused by infection with the germ *Mycobacterium avium,* has been eradicated from commercial chicken flocks, but still pops up occasionally in backyard chicken flocks. Because the avian TB organisms live in soil and water as well as in animals, birds aren't the most common source of infection for people who contract avian TB.

Healthy people are highly resistant to infection with *Mycobacterium avium,* but people whose immune systems are weakened by HIV infection or cancer are at high risk of becoming infected and developing severe disease. Avian TB is extremely difficult to treat with the drugs that are currently available.

✔ **Parrot fever:** Of domesticated poultry, turkeys are the most common carriers of parrot fever bacteria, but a few confirmed chicken cases have been reported. Compared to other birds, chickens are quite resistant to infection with parrot fever bacteria, and if they do become infected, they rarely show any signs of illness. You're much more likely to catch parrot fever from a parrot, parakeet, or pigeon than from a backyard chicken.

People who get parrot fever, also referred to as *psittacosis* or *avian chlamydiosis,* usually think they have the flu. The course of parrot fever typically runs ten days, and signs include fever, headache, chills, weakness, and coughing. Sometimes the infection is serious enough to put a person in the hospital, and deaths due to parrot fever have occurred. Tetracycline antibiotics are used to treat both human and bird infections.

Using Common Sense to Protect Yourself

Although this chapter lists some scary diseases, we don't suggest that you give up raising chickens. No hobby (or part-time job, for some small flock keepers) is risk-free, and if you put it in perspective, the risks and consequences of a healthy person contracting a disease from a chicken are low. With some common-sense precautions, you can reduce the risks to yourself and your family of picking up a disease from a backyard chicken.

Here is a disgustingly simple way to think about protecting people from important chicken-transmitted diseases: It's all about keeping chicken poop out of people's mouths. Gross, but true.

- ✔ **Supervise small children around chicks.** Kids, especially those under age 5, can't resist kissing those cute little fluffballs. Teach them not to, and make sure that they wash their hands after playing with chicks or touching chickens.

- ✔ **Everyone should wash their hands with soap and water after handling chickens and doing chicken chores.** Use alcohol hand sanitizer only if you don't have immediate access to soap and water.

- ✔ **Don't eat or drink around your chickens.** Keep live chickens out of the kitchen and off food preparation surfaces, and don't wash poultry equipment, such as feeders, waterers, and transport coops, in the kitchen sink.

- ✔ **Clean household items (like your favorite coffee cup left on the garden bench) that chickens have investigated and contaminated.** Wash them in the dishwasher or by hand with hot soapy water before using them again.

- ✔ **Don't eat raw eggs or undercooked poultry meat, even if you raised it.** See Chapter 20 for safe poultry product preparation. Don't feed raw eggs or undercooked meat to your chickens.

- ✔ **Keep your chickens clean, comfortable, and well fed to prevent disease in the flock.** Refer to Chapters 4, 5, and 6. Control rodents and do what you can to keep wild birds from hanging out with your flock.

- ✔ **Open doors and windows to increase ventilation when you're cleaning the coop.** Spray down dusty surfaces with water before sweeping or wiping them. If you must work in a dusty coop or closed-up poultry house, wear a dust mask, which you can purchase at hardware stores.

Chapter 20

Food Safety and Quality of Homegrown Eggs and Meat

In This Chapter
▶ Knowing how to handle eggs
▶ Understanding the importance of quality and food safety when processing your chickens

Chickens routinely carry two very common bacterial infections that cause food poisoning in people. *Salmonella* and *Campylobacter* bacteria are two chicken-associated germs that are usually transmitted to people by the *fecal-oral route*, meaning that people have to get chicken droppings (even microscopic amounts) in their mouths in order to come down with the infections. Chapter 19 discusses these bacteria in more depth and includes some simple and disgusting advice: Avoid eating chicken poop, and you avoid the most important chicken-transmitted infections.

In this chapter, we take that revolting idea a step further. Food safety, for a backyard flock keeper, is all about keeping chicken poop out of food — in this case, homegrown eggs and meat. Bon appetit!

Properly Handling Eggs

A good egg is a clean egg, and clean eggs start with a clean environment for your layers. Some dirty eggs are inevitable, however, so we share secrets on dry cleaning and washing eggs properly. No matter if you're enjoying an ultra-fresh omelet, keeping your egg customers happy, or successfully hatching lots of healthy chicks, the following advice applies to you.

Managing layers and nests

One of the best ways to reduce disease in your eggs is to keep an eye on your hens and their nests. When doing so, strive for eggs that are clean, straight out of the nest. That's not an easy feat for flock keepers with playful free-range hens who hide eggs in strange places and run through mud puddles, chasing tasty worm treats. Here are some tips to help you improve your daily clean egg collection rate:

- ✔ **Confine the flock to a fenced area.** Doing so can discourage hens from hiding eggs or nesting any place they have the urge.

- ✔ **Keep the layers' environment clean and dry.** Make sure the hens' yard has good drainage in rainy weather. Pay attention to the area around coop entrances, because these areas are prone to becoming muddy. Spread straw, wood shavings, or gravel in those places to keep mud to a minimum.

- ✔ **Control pests.** Keep *Salmonella*-spreading rats, mice, snakes, and flies out of the layers' living space.

- ✔ **Supply one nest box for every four to five hens in the flock.** Metal or plastic nest boxes are much easier to clean and less likely to harbor mites and lice than wooden nest boxes.

- ✔ **Make sure roosts are higher than the nest boxes.** Hens like to sleep off the ground on the highest roosts they can find. Placing the roosts higher can prevent hens from sleeping in the boxes and pooping in them.

- ✔ **Keep nest boxes bedded deeply with clean, dry nest material, such as straw or shavings.** Clean out the nest boxes and replace the bedding when it gets wet or dirty, or at least every two weeks.

- ✔ **Collect eggs twice a day in nice weather, and more often if the weather is freezing or hot.** Use collection containers that are easy to clean, such as coated wire baskets or plastic egg flats. Regularly clean and disinfect the containers; you can let the dishwasher do the work of sanitizing egg baskets or flats.

Most hens lay their eggs in the morning before 10 a.m., and they rarely lay after 3 p.m.

To wash or not to wash?

To answer that non-rhetorical question, we should expound on an amazing feature of eggs: germ-resistant packaging.

A hen provides excellent customer service, shining and polishing her eggs with a protective coating before delivering them to you. The waxy *cuticle,* also called *bloom,* is applied to the eggshell at the last station in the hen's oviduct. The cuticle has natural antibacterial activity and, along with the shell and shell membranes, it physically blocks germs from entering the egg. The cuticle, shell, and shell membranes don't make an impenetrable force field; germs teeming on the outside of a filthy egg can overwhelm the egg's natural barriers and get inside.

Avoid cleaning clean-looking eggs because cleaning disrupts the natural protective cuticle of the egg. You're better off cleaning dirty eggs if you want to keep them to eat or hatch. Dry cleaning is usually sufficient for lightly soiled eggs, but you must wash or discard very dirty eggs. Clean the dirty eggs as soon after gathering them as possible and definitely before you put them in the refrigerator.

Dry cleaning

No, we don't mean you take your eggs to the dry cleaners with your laundry. You can dry clean lightly soiled eggs by rubbing them with something mildly abrasive, such as a dry wash cloth, egg brush, sanding sponge, loofa, or even fine grit sandpaper. Clean and disinfect your egg cleaning tools regularly (or discard and replace them).

Washing

The best and safest way to wash eggs is with an expensive egg washing machine, which isn't an option for most small backyard flock keepers. If you don't have a washing machine, you can try this practical, food-safety savvy technique for hand washing your eggs.

You can use the washing technique that we suggest for eggs you, your family, and your guests eat, but not eggs offered for sale to the public. Small flock keepers in the United States who sell their eggs should check with their state's department of agriculture for rules about processing eggs for sale. (See the sidebar "Selling eggs from a backyard flock: Know the rules.")

You need: a clean one-gallon watering can, a clean sink with plenty of potable water, a roll of paper towels, and a trash can or compost bucket for used paper towels and discarded eggs. You also need a food-grade detergent and sanitizer. You can purchase a commercial FDA-approved egg wash product, or you can use unscented dishwashing detergent and regular strength household bleach.

Here's where we fly in the face of conventional wisdom (and current USDA rules requiring commercial egg processors to use warm water for washing eggs). We suggest using cool water, instead of warm or hot water, for washing and rinsing eggs for two main reasons:

- ✔ Cooling eggs as quickly as possible reduces the chance that *Salmonella* bacteria inside an egg will multiply.

- ✔ Warm water can create thermal cracks in an egg that open the door for germs to invade the egg.

Follow these easy steps for washing your eggs that you intend to eat:

1. **Fill the watering can with one gallon of cool tap water.**

2. **To the water in the can, add a small amount of dishwashing detergent and one tablespoon of regular strength household bleach.**

   You can also use the commercial egg wash product according to the directions on the label.

3. **Leave the eggs in a coated wire basket, plastic egg flat, or a colander, and set them in the sink.**

4. **Sprinkle the eggs with plenty of wash solution from the watering can.**

   Make sure the wash water goes down the drain; *never* let the eggs soak in water, especially dirty water.

5. **Let the eggs sit for 1 to 2 minutes.**

   Very dirty eggs may need a repeat flush from the watering can.

6. **Take each egg and wipe it with a new paper towel.**

   You can dip a new paper towel in the wash solution to wet and wipe an egg, but don't put a used towel in the wash solution or reuse a towel on another egg.

7. **Put the washed eggs in a different clean basket or egg flat.**

8. **Rinse the eggs with plenty of clean, cool tap water.**

9. **Put the washed and rinsed eggs, still in their basket or flat, in the refrigerator to chill and air dry.**

   You can sort and pack the washed eggs into clean cartons after they're dry.

Washing an egg improperly can turn one egg that's dirty on the outside into a whole basket of eggs that are dirty on the inside, too. A washed egg spoils sooner than an unwashed egg, because removing the egg's protective coating allows air, moisture, and germs to penetrate the shell more easily. Clean, intact, unwashed eggs have a shelf life of 30 days at room temperature. (In fact, most egg consumers around the world purchase eggs that have never been refrigerated.) Washed eggs, on the other hand, won't fare as well sitting out on the counter, and you should refrigerate them promptly.

Inspecting and storing eggs

Sort and inspect eggs before you store, eat, or sell them. Fresh eggs with minor cracks or shell imperfections like ridges, weird shapes, or thin spots are edible if you cook these eggs thoroughly and eat them right away. Don't sell oddball or cracked eggs to your customers though, because they break easily and most of your customers won't like the looks of them.

You can use a bright light to *candle* eggs and reveal minor cracks or eggs with undesirable blood spots inside (blood spots are edible, but they're a turn-off for your customers). A hand-held LED flashlight works very well for candling small batches of eggs. In the United States, your local extension office can refer you to publications about how to candle eggs to determine interior quality, including www.caes.uga.edu/extension/lumplin/4H/documents/EggsInt.Ext.pdf.

Egg grading is a method of inspecting and classifying the quality of an egg. Candling is an important part of the process of grading eggs. If you want to discover more about how to grade your eggs, check out the USDA Egg-Grading Manual, available at http://www.ams.usda.gov/AMSv1.0/getfile?dDocName=STELDEV3004502.

Although clean, unwashed eggs can sit on the kitchen countertop at room temperature for a couple of weeks and still taste good, we recommend putting clean, unwashed eggs in the refrigerator as soon as possible after collecting them, because *Salmonella* bacteria grow slower at cooler temperatures. You should immediately refrigerate washed eggs after washing them. Here are a few more egg storage tips and some preparation advice:

- ✔ **Store eggs large end up in the main part of the refrigerator.** Don't store them in the door, where the eggs are shaken and the temperature swings up and down. Don't store them near smelly foods like onions or fish because eggs can pick up odors.

- ✔ **Keep whole eggs about six to eight weeks in the refrigerator.** We're sure that eating old, musty eggs isn't one of the reasons that you keep chickens, so we don't suggest keeping the eggs much longer.

- ✔ **You can freeze eggs.** Crack them and separate egg whites and yolks into different containers before putting the containers into the freezer. Frozen egg whites or yolks will keep indefinitely, and typically are still tasty after storage for up to a year in the freezer.

- ✔ **Date your egg cartons.** Use your two- to three-week old eggs for hard-boiling, because fresher eggs are harder to peel.

- ✔ **Cook eggs until the yolks are firm.** Unless you're a healthy, consenting adult willing to take your chances with *Salmonella,* don't eat raw eggs, even if they came straight from your own healthy hens. If you're pregnant, never eat raw eggs.

Selling eggs from a backyard flock: Know the rules

In most U.S. states, you can legally sell eggs from your small home flock (of less than 3,000 hens) directly to consumers without a license and without inspection. Check with your state's department of agriculture to find out the rules, which are intended to protect the public from foodborne illnesses.

Where you live, rules for selling eggs may specify:

✔ **Acceptable egg cartons:** You may be required to use new cartons, or in some places, reused but clean cartons are okay.

✔ **Required labeling:** You may be required to label the carton with your name, contact information, and other details about your eggs.

✔ **Processing conditions:** Clean, unwashed eggs may be okay, or you may be required to wash them. You probably won't be required to candle and grade your eggs.

✔ **Storage conditions:** Egg sales regulations may specify the temperature at which you must store your eggs until they're put in your customer's hands.

Producing Safe, High Quality Meat from Your Own Flock

This section focuses on the food safety aspects of processing chickens at home, rather than providing a complete tutorial on butchering chickens. You can find those instructions elsewhere, such as in *Raising Chickens For Dummies* by Kimberly Willis and Rob Ludlow (John Wiley & Sons, Inc.) or in a number of cooperative extension service publications. Use the following tips to produce safe, high-quality meat for your family and guests. If you process homegrown chickens with attention to detail, we believe your product can match or exceed commercial processing conditions for cleanliness and quality.

Choosing and preparing your birds

When you select your own chickens to process at home, make sure you keep stress for the birds to a minimum prior to butchering. You have the advantage that the birds don't need to be trucked many miles from your farm to a processing plant, and you can take your time, handling the birds gently and quietly.

Stress causes chickens that are carrying *Salmonella* or *Campylobacter* bacteria in their intestinal tracts to shed more of the germs in their droppings. Rough handling and heat stress can also toughen meat, so reducing stress is not just an animal welfare issue, but it's also an important food safety and meat quality issue.

Here are other best practices for choosing and preparing poultry for slaughter:

- ✔ **Choose birds that appear healthy and that are in good body condition.** You should feel plenty of flesh over the *keel* (breastbone) of each bird.

- ✔ **Avoid processing birds with lots of pinfeathers.** Plucking these feathers is frustrating and time consuming. Wait a couple of weeks until the feathers grow in.

- ✔ **Fast (don't feed) birds for six to eight hours before slaughter, but always keep water available to them.** Fasting empties the gut and reduces the chance of fecal contamination of the carcass.

- ✔ **Hold birds in a wire-bottomed cage during fasting.** Droppings fall through the wire floor, which helps to keep the caged birds clean.

Don't ever process cadavers for human consumption! A *cadaver* is a bird that died for any reason other than being intentionally slaughtered for food. Don't process them, regardless of the reason you think the bird may have died, because it's not safe.

Preparing the work area

Your processing area should be clean, as fly-free as possible, and have plenty of clean, running water. Separate the area into a place for very dirty jobs (killing, scalding, and plucking), and a place for less dirty jobs (gutting, inspecting, chilling, and packaging). Start with clean tools, surfaces, and hands.

Spread a new disposable plastic tablecloth (a dollar store item) on your work table to give yourself a sanitary surface and easy cleanup when you're done processing. Bag the tablecloth when you're finished, along with any used disposable gloves and paper towels, and dispose of them with the household trash in a receptacle with a scavenger-proof lid.

Sanitizing between birds

Before you actually start to butcher any chickens, you first need to prepare a sanitizing solution to use in the processing area. To mix and use the sanitizer solution during processing, follow these simple steps:

1. **Add one tablespoon of regular strength household bleach to a one-gallon watering can full of clean water.**

2. **Use the solution to fill a pan to soak your tools in between birds.**

3. **Sprinkle the table with the solution and wipe it down with a fresh paper towel after you're finished *eviscerating* (gutting) each bird.**

   Using the watering can is a trick to remind you to keep the solution clean; you can easily forget and dunk your dirty tools in your stock batch of sanitizer, if it's in a bucket.

Inspecting your processed chickens

After you have killed, scalded, and plucked the bird, you have to decide if it's a keeper. (Not to worry — a chicken that appeared healthy prior to slaughter rarely fails the postmortem inspection.) As you gut the bird, take a minute or two to perform a simple inspection. Here are the steps:

1. **Look at the outside of the bird.**

   The skin should be free of tumors, large bruises, or big areas of discoloration. You can trim off small bruises or skin defects.

2. **Check the general body condition.**

   A healthy bird has plenty of flesh covering the keel. The breast muscle should look pale compared to the muscles of the thigh and drumstick.

3. **Check for symmetry.**

   The legs, wings, and sides of the breast should look symmetrical.

4. **Peek inside.**

   As you open the body cavity to gut the bird, look for fluid inside the cavity. The insides of a healthy bird are moist, but shouldn't have more than a trace of free fluid. A well-fed bird has lots of bright yellow abdominal fat, which is normal.

5. **Examine the abdominal organs as you remove them.**

   After processing a few birds, you can get used to what's normal. Examine the liver surface and check the texture by gently pressing with your fingers. The liver should be smooth and uniformly colored, and it shouldn't fall apart in your hands. Take a quick look at the color and texture of the other innards.

Passing judgment

Finding something odd during your inspection may indicate a problem that is benign, but unappetizing. It may be a true health hazard — you won't be able to tell for certain with your brief visual inspection. Our philosophy is that you're better safe than sorry (or disappointed at the dinner table after doing all that work), so we recommend that you reject any chicken carcass with these signs or conditions:

- ✔ Lumps or spots of any size on the surface of the liver.

- ✔ More than a trace of fluid in the body cavity.

- ✔ Small red or purple round spots *(petechiae)* on the surface of more than one internal organ.

- ✔ Any individual internal organ that's two or more times the normal size (compare the organ with another from a bird of similar size). Ignore gall bladder size, which can vary a lot, in this observation.

- ✔ Breast meat with the same coloration as the meat of the thighs and legs.

- ✔ Meat showing white streaks or an area of abnormal enlargement when compared to the same area on the opposite side of the bird.

Chillin' the chicken

Chilling the carcasses as quickly as possible after slaughter is very important to prevent the growth of bacteria that cause foodborne illness. Challenge yourself to get the chicken chilled to 40 degrees Fahrenheit (4 degrees Celsius) within four hours of slaughter. You can make it easily, if you don't get hung up by a bunch of pinfeathers, and it gets easier to beat your personal best chill time as you gain experience at processing.

Immersing the processed chickens in lots of ice and plenty of clean, cold running water is the secret to a quick chill. Sturdy 70 quart muck buckets with rope handles make great chill tanks for home use (without the muck). Let the garden hose run continuously into your chill tank with a small stream of cold water. After the chickens are icy cold (it should take an hour or two, depending on the size of the birds), you can package and put them in the refrigerator.

Preparing and storing the meat

You're now ready to enjoy a truly homemade chicken dinner. Cook chicken thoroughly to an internal temperature of at least 165 degrees F (74 degrees C).

If you processed a large batch of birds, you can save some for later. Stored poultry stays flavorful and wholesome if you follow these tips:

✔ **Age freshly processed chicken in the refrigerator as a tenderizing technique.** Allow fresh chicken to rest in the refrigerator for one to five days before cooking or freezing it for more tender meat.

✔ **Freshly processed chickens can stay in the refrigerator for no more than five days.** You need to eat them or freeze them before then.

✔ **Don't freeze a lot of fresh processed birds at once.** Trying to freeze a large amount of fresh meat can take a long time, and in the meantime, other things in the freezer may warm up and start to thaw. Freeze a few birds at a time, leaving a little space between each bird. You can stack them closer after they're all frozen solid.

✔ **You can keep poultry frozen for a year, but the meat will taste better if you use it within six to eight months of freezing.** To thaw a frozen chicken, put it in the refrigerator for 24 to 48 hours; don't thaw meat at room temperature. (If you need to thaw it faster, use cold, running water or a microwave.)

Part VI
The Part of Tens

The 5th Wave   By Rich Tennant

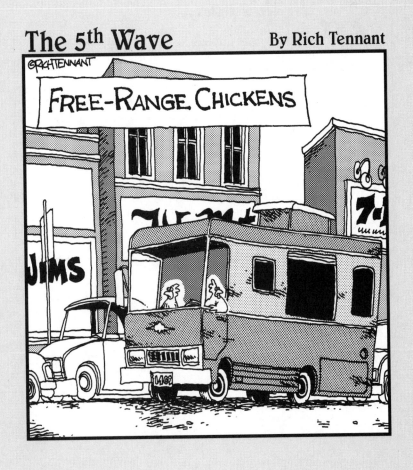

In this part...

When people find out that you're a small flock keeper, some of them probably ask you how to keep a flock healthy, especially if they're new to flock keeping or considering getting chickens. We hope the two chapters in this part make it easier for you to be an ambassador for backyard chickens. You can use the brief answers to some of the most common questions about chicken health and dispel the most common misconceptions.

Finally, in the appendix, you can find recipes for home remedies we mention elsewhere in the book, and refer to a guide about the pros and cons of disinfectants for good flock keeping.

Chapter 21

Answers to Ten Common Questions about Chicken Health

In This Chapter

▶ Finding quick answers to common questions about alarming chicken health issues

▶ Getting and giving concise advice on chicken care do's and don'ts

*I*n this chapter, we assemble the most common questions that we hear flock keepers ask about the health of their chickens. We provide quick, concise answers that you can take to heart or share with a fellow flock keeper in the time it takes you to check out at the feed store.

What Is That Lump on the Side of My Chicken's Neck?

Most likely, the lump on the side of your chicken's neck is normal. That's her *crop,* an expandable pouch in the esophagus of chickens and many other types of birds that is part of the digestive system. Think of that anatomical feature as a doggie bag — a place for the foraging hen to store her edible discoveries for digestion sometime later in the day.

Rarely, a chicken's crop plugs up because she's eaten a lot of indigestible stuff, such as straw, wood chips, or long, stemmy weeds (we don't know why she swallows that stuff). The condition is known as a *crop impaction,* and it can be serious. (See Chapter 14 for prevention tips.) If you're concerned that the hard lump may be an impaction, feel the chicken's neck early the next morning, before she has eaten breakfast. The lump should be gone, and her throat should feel soft and empty.

Why Is My Chicken Losing Her Feathers?

Molt happens. Each year, usually in autumn, a chicken loses her old feathers and grows a new set, in an orderly process called *molting*. Most hens slow down on egg production or quit laying eggs altogether while they're molting. Some hens molt quickly and get it over with in two to three months, although others can take as long as six months to freshen their appearance. If your chicken is losing her feathers, suspect molt first.

Other common causes of feather loss include *feather pecking* (flock mates are plucking out feathers) and external parasites (mites or lice, usually). You may be able to blame the hens' bare backs on the rooster's attention — he's scratching feathers out during mating. (If you have bare-backed hens and no rooster, a dominant hen is probably stepping in to fill the rooster's role.) We cover feather loss in more detail in Chapter 8.

Why Do Some Eggs Have Soft Shells or No Shells?

Stress is the number-one cause of abnormal eggshells in hens, including soft or shell-less eggs. Events that stress hens are disturbances that are likely to bother you, too; moving to a new home, meeting a guest's rambunctious dog or child, hot weather, or a sudden and violent storm are common stressors. A single disturbance can affect a flock's egg production for a couple of weeks.

Besides stress, other explanations may fit. Older hens and hens that have been *in lay* (producing eggs) for many months are more likely to lay soft-shelled eggs. Viral infections can also mess up a hen's egg-laying machinery, sometimes permanently. See Chapter 8 for details.

How Do I Treat My Chicken's Skin Wounds?

The most common backyard chicken wounds are the result of predator attacks, flock-mate aggression, and entanglement or impalement by something sharp in the chicken yard, such as broken wire fences or protruding nails.

Here are a few tips for immediate care of injured chickens:

1. **Treat predator bite wounds and other skin wounds as soon as you discover them.**

   Wounds inflicted by cats, in particular, are highly likely to become infected, and prompt treatment may avert a life-threatening wound infection.

2. **Thoroughly flush the wound with an antiseptic solution.**

   We describe the procedure in detail in Chapter 17, and give an easy recipe for a dilute Dakin's antiseptic solution in the appendix.

3. **Isolate the injured bird from the rest of the flock and let her take care of the wound herself.**

   Don't slather the wound with ointments or stitch the wound yourself. Most skin wounds should be left open; talk to a vet if you're not sure.

4. **Talk to your veterinarian before medicating a chicken with an antibiotic.**

What Causes My Chicken to Have Runny Poop?

Having loose droppings can be normal if they're intermittent with normal, formed poop. Two or three times a day, a chicken empties the contents of the *ceca,* which are two blind pouches in the lower part of the digestive system. The cecal droppings are loose, brown, very smelly, and completely normal for chickens.

If all the chicken's droppings are runny, however, that's abnormal, so look for a health problem. Heading the list of possibilities for adult bird diarrhea is hot weather, which is a very common reason for laying hens to have loose droppings. Take this sign as a warning to ease the flock's heat stress. Suspect the parasitic disease *coccidiosis* anytime a young chicken has runny poop (see Chapter 13 for prevention and treatment of coccidiosis). A veterinary diagnostic lab can help you find the cause for chicken diarrhea.

Should I Feed My Chicks Medicated Starter Feed?

Yes, we think you should feed your chicks medicated starter feed, except under two conditions, which we get to later. First, we should give you a quick rundown on the purpose of medicated chick starter feed.

The medication in medicated chick starter is a *coccidiostat,* a drug that helps prevent coccidiosis. We describe coccidiosis in more detail in Chapter 13, but put simply, a parasite that lives wherever chickens are raised causes the extremely common chick-killing disease. Before the invention of coccidiostats, raising chicks without losing some to coccidiosis was a big challenge for flock keepers.

Approved coccidiostats, such as amprolium, are mixed into the feed at a low dose and given to chicks from hatch day until they're about 4 months old. (The label indicates how to use the medicated feed; carefully follow the label directions for best results.) Used according to label directions, coccidiostats are very safe, both for the chicks and the people who eventually consume eggs or meat from the treated chicks. The low dose of medication doesn't eliminate all the coccidia parasites, but it keeps them down to a dull roar while the chicks develop some natural immunity to the parasites.

Don't use medicated starter feed if either of two situations applies to your chicks:

- ✔ **Your chicks were vaccinated for coccidiosis.** Some hatcheries vaccinate your mail-order chicks for coccidiosis at your request. Feeding medicated starter feed to vaccinated chicks defeats the purpose of the vaccination.

- ✔ **You're trying to raise chickens under organic conditions.** Coccidiosis vaccination may be a good option for you, instead of medicated feed.

I Gave My Hen Medicine. Is It Safe for Me to Eat Her Eggs?

Any medication given to a laying hen can end up in the eggs that she produces, sometimes for several weeks after being dosed. Very few medications have been studied thoroughly to determine how long they'll contaminate the eggs of medicated hens, and therefore, very few medications have been approved for use in laying hens.

Antibiotics, dewormers, and anti-inflammatories are medications that backyard flock keepers often want to use to help their hens feel better. Many of these drugs are also used in human medicine, and serious adverse reactions are rare for people receiving these drugs. However, we can't tell you that eggs from medicated hens are completely safe for personal consumption; it wouldn't be ethical or legal. Although we can't help in this case, your veterinarian can, if you discuss the drug, dose, and duration you used to medicate the chicken. Here's our advice when it comes to medicating laying hens:

✔ Avoid giving laying hens medication of any kind.

✔ Talk to a veterinarian if you think you need to medicate laying hens. Your veterinarian can help you make a diagnosis, and if medication is appropriate, provide you with a prescription and an egg discard time.

✔ If you become aware that a hen was inadvertently medicated without a prescription, consult a vet or discard the medicated hen's eggs for at least eight weeks after the last dose.

What Are These Bugs Crawling on My Bird (and Me)?

They're lice or mites, almost certainly. These extremely common external parasites feed on your chickens, irritating and weakening them. Lice and mites can crawl on you, too, if you handle infested birds. Although chicken lice think people taste disgusting (they won't hang around for long), mites will happily bite a person before running back to their preferred host — your chicken. Chapter 13 has ways to deal with these tiny terrors.

What Is Causing My Hen's Swollen Foot and Her Limping?

Bumblefoot is a common infection of the feet of poultry, usually discovered as a swollen, scabby foot pad. The problem starts with minor trauma to the foot, such as a bruise, scrape, cut, or puncture. Bacteria invade the small foot wound and create a big mess, causing pus-filled abscesses, swelling, and pain. Treatment isn't quick or easy, and it usually requires repeated draining and cleaning the wound. See Chapter 14 for bumblefoot prevention and treatment advice.

Can I Feed Bugs and Worms to My Flock?

We think bugs and worms are yummy and nutritious (for your chickens). A chicken isn't a vegetarian by nature, and she relishes a nice, juicy bug, which is typically loaded with nutritious fat and protein.

Although insects and worms can harbor and transmit internal parasites, such as tapeworms, the risk is low to chickens if the insects and worms that you feed weren't raised in a chicken yard or otherwise exposed to chicken poop, because chickens and their droppings are a necessary part of the lifecycle of the parasites. Packaged mealworms, black soldier grubs grown in kitchen compost, and earthworms dug from the vegetable garden are relatively safe treats that can make your chickens adore you.

Chapter 22

Ten Common Misconceptions about Chicken Health and Treatments

*I*n this chapter, we list ten of the most famous backyard flock-keeping myths. By busting these myths, we may burst some bubbles of wishful thinking, but hopefully, we also ease some unnecessary worries.

Mixing a New, Healthy-Looking Chicken with the Flock Is Safe

Many types of organisms that cause diseases in chickens can live hidden within a chicken, causing no signs of illness, or causing signs that are so mild that no one notices them. A healthy-looking carrier chicken can harbor a disease-causing organism for a long time, often the rest of her life, and she may spread the infection to flock mates without anyone being aware of it. You take a risk of introducing disease anytime you bring a new chicken home, especially an adult chicken, who has been alive long enough to pick up who-knows-what.

You Can Get Worms from Eating Eggs from Wormy Hens

Intestinal worms are so common in free-range chickens that we'd have a big public-health problem on our hands if this myth were true. You don't need to worry about getting worms from wormy chickens. Intestinal worms are fairly fussy about whose intestines they live in, so chicken worms don't like to set up residence in people.

Occasionally, a wormy hen can lay an egg with a worm inside, but that's just a revolting surprise at breakfast, not a human health hazard.

You Can Use Horse or Dog Medicine for Chickens

Giving a chicken a medication that isn't labeled for use in chickens is called *extra-label drug use,* and it's illegal in the United States unless a licensed veterinarian who knows you and your flock prescribes the medication. To stay on the right side of food safety rules, use over-the-counter medications only as directed on the label, or consult a veterinarian.

Many Medicines Are Approved for Use in Laying Hens

We wish this misconception were true! Very few medications are approved for use in chickens producing eggs for human consumption. You may suspect that drugs fail to win approval because they're unsafe or they have side effects for hens, but that's rarely the snag in the process. Mostly, the holdup is because veterinary drug makers haven't found it worthwhile to spend time and money on the extensive research that's required to prove that eggs from treated chickens are safe for people to eat.

Natural Remedies Are Always Safer Than Synthetic Drugs

People who recommend or sell natural remedies aren't required to prove that those remedies are safe or effective, so we don't know much about the safety and efficacy of many substances touted as natural cures. Calling a substance *natural* doesn't guarantee its safety (snake venom is natural!). Virtually everything, even water, has a toxic dose.

We know for sure that some natural remedies aren't very safe. For example, tobacco is an old-time natural remedy for chicken intestinal worms. The nicotine in tobacco leaves will kill some worms, no doubt; however, it's a tossup whether it will poison the chicken first. A number of synthetic dewormers are many times safer and more effective than that particular natural remedy.

Vaccinating Is the Best Way to Prevent Flock Infections

In general, poultry vaccines are a better tool for managing a disease that is already affecting a flock than they are at keeping disease out. The best way to prevent an infection from entering a flock is through good biosecurity. Keeping a closed flock and not sharing poultry equipment with other flock keepers are just two of many biosecurity measures that are probably more effective than vaccination in preventing flock infections. See Chapter 4 for tips on developing your own biosecurity plan.

Surgery Will Stop Your Rooster from Crowing

Successful decrowing surgery would be a life-saving procedure for many urban and suburban roosters (and welcome relief to their neighbors). Unfortunately, no foolproof procedure exists that reliably stops a live rooster from crowing. The rooster's voice box (the *syrinx*) is located deep inside his chest, close to the heart — a tricky place to operate.

You Must Regularly Deworm and Vaccinate Backyard Flocks

Almost all backyard chickens carry a few intestinal worms, which don't usually cause a problem (actually, having a few worms may boost the immune system). We don't suggest regular, routine deworming for backyard chickens, unless you know you have a parasite problem in your flock. We feel the same about vaccinations, because chicken shots are more effective at controlling disease than preventing flock infections. Most backyard flock keepers can help their flock more by focusing on biosecurity and keeping the flock clean, comfortable, and well fed rather than spending time and money on routine vaccinations.

Chickens Catch Colds, and They Recover in a Few Days

Chickens catch respiratory infections that cause signs similar to human colds, but the chicken cold germs aren't the same as the cold germs that afflict people. The big problem with several germs that cause chicken colds is that they never go away — chickens can become permanent carriers (and spreaders) of the germ after they become infected, even if they appear to get over it in a few days.

A Hen That Eats Her Eggs Has a Nutritional Deficiency

Egg-eating is an infuriating habit that some laying hens pick up. Even pampered, well-fed birds can become intractable egg-eaters; poor nutrition is rarely to blame. The egg-eating habit is nearly impossible to break after a chicken starts doing it, and she often recruits other flock members in her crime spree.

Although egg-eater rehab programs are rarely successful, prevention works. You can prevent egg-eating by reducing the chances of egg breakage: Collect eggs frequently, don't scare hens, and keep plenty of protective padding, such as straw, shavings, or artificial turf, in the nest boxes.

Appendix

Chicken Health Formulary

⬤ ⬤

*I*n this appendix, we stow the details for coop disinfectants and the medication recipes that we refer to in other parts of this book.

Read the label before you buy a disinfectant or medication for your flock to make sure it's the right stuff for your job, and read the label again before you use the product. Follow the directions on the label, which spell out how to mix, store, use, and dispose of the product safely.

Flock keepers can use medications for their chickens according to label directions. Using a drug, such as an antibiotic or dewormer, in a way that isn't listed on the label (a different dose, or different type of animal, for example) is *extra-label use,* which is against the law in the United States unless you have a prescription from a veterinarian. See Chapter 16 for more information about medicating chickens.

Disinfectants for Poultry Premises

Table A-1 lists common types of disinfectants used on poultry premises, gives examples of each type, and cites the main advantages and disadvantages.

Table A-1	Characteristics of Disinfectants			
Type	**Examples**	**Best Used For**	**Main Advantage**	**Main Disadvantage**
Alcohols	Hand sanitizers, rubbing alcohol	Hands and small objects	Works quickly	No residual activity
Aldehydes	Gluteraldehyde	Sanitizing surfaces and small objects	Broad-spectrum germ killers	Irritating to skin, eyes, and respiratory tract
Iodines or chlorines	Povidone-iodine, household bleach, chlorine dioxide	Sanitizing surfaces and small objects	Broad-spectrum germ killers	Inactivated by organic matter (dirt)
Organic acids	Citric acid, vinegar	Sanitizing surfaces and small objects	Removes mineral deposits	Not very effective at low temperatures
Oxidizing agents	Hydrogen peroxide, peracetic acid, Virkon-S	Sanitizing surfaces and small objects	Not inactivated by organic matter	Corrodes some types of metal
Phenolics	Phenol	Surfaces	Not inactivated by organic matter	Irritating, smelly, and corrosive
Quaternary ammonium	Roccal-D and other *quats*	Cleaning incubators and brooders	Non-irritating and low toxicity	Inactivated by soap

Medication Solutions for Backyard Flocks

You may already have a well-stocked backyard flock medicine cabinet. Table A-2 lists some inexpensive solutions that you can make at home from common ingredients or items you can pick up at most pharmacies or hardware stores.

Table A-2   Home Remedies for Backyard Chickens

Medication	Purpose	Solution Preparation	How to Use the Solution
Aspirin drinking-water solution	Ease pain and inflammation from injury, egg peritonitis, or gout	Crush five 325 mg (5 grain) aspirin tablets and dissolve in 1 gallon of water.	Provide solution as the only source of drinking water for the bird for 1 to 3 days.
Boric acid eye wash	Cleaning eyes, treating conjunctivitis	Purchase boric acid powder at a pharmacy. Mix ¼ teaspoon of boric acid powder into 1 cup of distilled water. Mix well and store in a clean bottle.	Wet a cotton ball and swab the eye one to two times daily for 3 days.
Chlorinated drinking water	Sanitize drinking water	Mix ⅛ teaspoon of household bleach with each gallon of drinking water.	Provide as the only source of drinking water. Okay to use continuously.
Copper sulfate solution	Treating thrush (also referred to as *candidiasis*), a yeast infection in the crop	Dissolve 1 ounce of copper sulfate and 1 tablespoon of vinegar in 15 gallons of water (or purchase acidified copper sulfate from a poultry-supply company and use according to label directions).	Provide solution as the only source of drinking water for the bird or flock for 3 days.
Dilute Dakin's solution	Flushing, cleaning, and daily treatment of skin wounds	Mix 1 tablespoon of household bleach and 1 teaspoon of baking soda in 1 gallon of distilled water. Cap and shake the jug to mix.	Flush the wound with the solution using a syringe, or swab the wound with gauze moistened with the solution.
Epsom salt drinking-water solution	Laxative to hasten elimination of toxins, including suspected botulism	Dissolve ⅓ cup of Epsom salts in each gallon of drinking water.	Provide solution as the only source of drinking water for the bird or flock for 1 day.

(continued)

Table A-2 *(continued)*

Medication	Purpose	Solution Preparation	How to Use the Solution
Iodine drinking-water solution	Supportive care for an outbreak of fowl pox	Mix 1 teaspoon of 1 percent iodine solution per gallon of water, or ½ half teaspoon of 2 percent iodine solution per gallon of water.	Provide as the only source of drinking water until outbreak subsides.
Vinegar drinking-water solution	Supportive care for diarrhea or thrush in the flock	Mix 2 tablespoons of vinegar with each gallon of drinking water.	Provide as the only source of drinking water for 1 week.
Vitamin C drinking-water solution	Supportive care for heat stress	Crush one 1,000 mg vitamin C tablet and add to each gallon of drinking water.	Provide as the only source of drinking water during periods of extremely hot weather. (Can combine with vitamin/electrolyte supplement.)

Parasite Treatments for Backyard Chickens

As we discuss in Chapter 13, internal and external parasites cause quite a bit of trouble for backyard chicken flocks. Table A-3 contains prevention and treatment for coccidiosis.

Table A-3 Coccidiosis Prevention and Treatment Options

Purpose	Option	Dose
Prevent coccidiosis outbreaks	Medicated chick starter	Use according to label directions.
	Coccidiosis vaccination	Ask the hatchery.
	Vinegar drinking-water solution	Mix 4 tablespoons of vinegar with each gallon of drinking water. Provide as the only source of drinking water.

Purpose	Option	Dose
Treat coccidio-sis outbreaks	Amprolium 9.6 percent solution	One teaspoon of amprolium solution per gallon of drinking water for 5 days; then ½ teaspoon per gallon of drinking water for 1 to 2 weeks. Double the dose for severe outbreaks. Okay for laying hens.
	Sulfadimethoxine or sulfamethazine 12.5 percent solution	Use according to label directions.

We don't recommend routine deworming for backyard flocks. First, find out if your birds have an intestinal parasite problem by consulting a veterinarian or veterinary diagnostic laboratory. We list four relatively safe and effective deworming options for chickens in Table A-4.

Table A-4   Intestinal Parasite Treatment Options

Option	Effective Against	Dose
Albendazole 11.36% suspension	Cecal worms, round-worms, tapeworms, threadworms	Consult a veterinarian before using for chickens intended to produce food for people. Give 0.1 cc per pound of chicken's weight by mouth. (Tip: use a 1 cc syringe.)
Fenbendazole 0.5% multi-species dewormer pellets	Cecal worms, gape-worms, roundworms, tapeworms, thread-worms	Consult a veterinarian before using for chickens intended to produce food for people. Feed ½ teaspoon of pellets for each pound of chicken's weight once a day for 3 days (about 1 tablespoon for each standard 5-pound hen).
Ivermectin 1% injectable solution	Cecal worms, round-worms, threadworms (also mites and lice)	Consult a veterinarian before using for chickens intended to produce food for people. Mix 2 cc (2 mL) with 1 gallon of drinking water. Provide as only source of drinking water for 2 days.
Piperazine 17% solution	Roundworms only	Consult a veterinarian before using for chickens intended to produce food for people. Use according to label directions.

Your chickens are likely to encounter external parasites. Table A-5 provides some practical small flock treatments for mites and lice.

Table A-5   External Parasite Treatment Options

Type	Purpose	Substance	Dose
Dustbath mixes	Chickens treat themselves to reduce mites and lice	Diatomaceous earth (DE)	50:50 mix (by volume) of DE and sand. Recharge bath once a month.
		Kaolin clay	50:50 mix (by volume) of kaolin clay and sand. Recharge bath once a month.
		90% sulfur powder	25:75 mix (by volume) of sulfur powder and sand. Recharge bath once a month.
Sprays or powders	Apply to chickens to reduce mites and lice	Pyrethrin or permethrin sprays or powders	Use according to label directions.
		10 percent garlic juice	Spray each hen, especially the vent area, once a week.
		70 percent neem oil	Mix 2 tablespoons of 70% neem oil with 1 gallon of water. Spray birds and coop once a week.
Ointments	Repel flies from wounds, control scaly leg mites	Petroleum jelly/ sulfur mix	Mix 2 tablespoons of sulfur powder with ½ cup of petroleum jelly. Apply to affected area daily until wound is healed or for at least 2 weeks for scaly leg mites.
	Control scaly leg mites	Ointment containing camphor	Apply a camphor ointment to affected bird's legs daily for at least 2 weeks.
Injectable or oral medication	Control serious louse or mite infestations, including scaly leg mites	Ivermectin	Obtain a prescription from a veterinarian. Give a 0.2 mg/kg dose of ivermectin to each bird; repeat in 10 days.

Index